THE GENETIC FRONTIER

ETHICS, LAW, AND POLICY

D1566233

THE GENETIC FRONTIER
ETHICS, LAW, AND POLICY

Mark S. Frankel and Albert H. Teich, Editors

Directorate for Science and Policy Programs
American Association for the
Advancement of Science

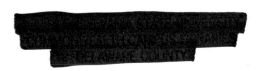

Copyright © 1994
American Association for the Advancement of Science
1333 H Street, NW, Washington, DC 20005 USA

Library of Congress Cataloging-in-Publication Data

The Genetic Frontier: ethics, law , and policy / Mark S. Frankel
and Albert H. Teich, editors.
        p. cm.
    Includes bibliographical references and index.
    ISBN 0-87168-526-4
    1. Medical genetics—Moral and ethical aspects.
    2. Medical ethics—Law and legislation.
    3. Medical genetics—Social aspects.
    I. Frankel, Mark S. II. Teich, Albert H. III.
    RB155.G3854
    174'.2—dc20   93-37230
                             CIP

AAAS Publication Number 93-27S
International Standard Book Number: 0-87168-526-4
Printed in the United States of America on acid-free, recycled paper

Table of Contents

Contributors   ix

Acknowledgments   xi

Introduction   xiii —
    Genetic Testing and the Human Genome Project
                 Albert H. Teich and Mark S. Frankel

Part I. Family Relationships and Social Policy

Introduction   3
    Genes and Families
                 Robert Mullan Cook-Deegan

Chapter 1   9 —
    Family Relationships and Social Policy:
    An Ethical Inquiry
                 Roger L. Shinn

Chapter 2   25
    And Baby Makes Three—Or Four, or Five, or Six:
    Defining the Family After the Genetic Revolution
                 R. Alta Charo

Part II. Privacy and Confidentiality Issues for Genetic Testing

Introduction   47 —
    Collection and Disclosure of Genetic Information
                 Laurence Tancredi

Chapter 3   53

    Privacy and Genetic Information:
    A Sociopolitical Analysis

                                      Alan F. Westin

Chapter 4   77

    Privacy and the Control of Genetic Information
                                  Madison Powers

Part III. Linking Genetics, Behavior, and Responsibility

Introduction   103

    Genetic and Environmental Influences on Behavior
                                    Alan I. Leshner

Chapter 5   105

    Genes, Behavior, and Responsibility:
    Research Perspectives

                                V. Elving Anderson

Chapter 6   131

    Human Genetics, Evolutionary Theory, and
    Social Stratification

                                     Troy Duster

Chapter 7   155

    Linking Genetics, Behavior, and Responsibility:
    Legal Implications

                                    Norval Morris

Chapter 8   161

    The Genetics of Moral Agency
                            Ronald S. Cole-Turner

Part IV. Genetic Testing and Determination of Property Rights

Introduction   177

    Scope and Value of Patent Protection
                                Gilbert S. Omenn

Chapter 9   181
    Intellectual Property and Genetic Testing
                              Kate H. Murashige

Chapter 10   199
    Intellectual Property and Genetic Testing:
    A Commentary
                              Thomas J. White

Chapter 11   209
    Intellectual Property and Genetic Testing:
    A Scientist's Perspective
                              Joan Overhauser

Chapter 12   215
    Intellectual Property and Human Dignity
                              Ted Peters

Appendix   225

Index   233

Contributors

V. Elving Anderson, Ph.D.
Professor Emeritus
Epilepsy Clinical Research Program
University of Minnesota
Minneapolis, MN

R. Alta Charo, J.D.
Professor of Law and Medical Ethics
University of Wisconsin Law School
Madison, WI

Ronald S. Cole-Turner, Ph.D, M.Div.
Associate Professor of Theology
Memphis Theological Seminary
Memphis, TN

Robert Mullan Cook-Deegan, M.D.
Director, Division of Biobehavioral
Sciences in Mental Disorders
Institute of Medicine
Derwood, MD

Troy Duster, Ph.D.
Director
Institute for the Study of Social
Change
University of California
Berkeley, CA

Mark S. Frankel, Ph.D.
Director
Scientific Freedom, Responsibility &
Law Program
Directorate for Science & Policy
Programs, AAAS
Washington, DC

Alan I. Leshner, Ph.D.
Deputy Director
National Institute of Mental Health
Rockville, MD

Norval Morris, J.D.
Professor of Law & Criminology
University of Chicago Law School
Chicago, IL

Kate Murashige, J.D., Ph.D.
Partner
Morrison & Foerster
Washington, DC

Gilbert S. Omenn, M.D., Ph.D.
Dean, School of Public Health &
Community Medicine
University of Washington
Seattle, WA

Joan Overhauser, Ph.D.
System Professor
Department of Biochemistry
& Molecular Biology
Thomas Jefferson University
Philadelphia, PA

Ted Peters, Ph.D., M.Div.
Professor of Systematic Theology
Center for Theology and
the Natural Sciences
Berkeley, CA

Madison Powers, Ph.D., J.D.
Senior Research Scholar
Kennedy Institute of Ethics
Assistant Professor of Philosophy
Georgetown University
Washington, D.C.

Roger Shinn, Ph.D., M.Div.
Reinhold Niebuhr Professor
Emeritus of Social Ethics
Union Theological Seminary
New York, NY

Laurence R. Tancredi, M.D., J.D.
Professor of Clinical Psychiatry
New York University
New York, NY

Albert H. Teich, Ph.D.
Director
Directorate for Science & Policy
Programs, AAAS
Washington, DC

Alan F. Westin, J.D., Ph.D.
Professor of Public Law &
Government
Department of Political Science
Columbia University
Teaneck, NJ

Thomas White, Ph.D.
Vice President for Research
& Development
Roche Molecular Systems
Alameda, CA

Acknowledgments

This book is the product of the last of three invitational conferences convened by the AAAS-American Bar Association National Conference of Lawyers and Scientists and the AAAS Committee on Scientific Freedom and Responsibility. The conference was held at Los Alamos National Laboratory, Los Alamos, New Mexico, in June 1992.

Many individuals and organizations contributed to the creation of this book. The members of the advisory committee to the AAAS Project on Ethical and Legal Implications of Genetic Testing provided overall guidance and direction to our efforts. The committee was chaired by Sheila Jasanoff and Ruth Greenstein; the names and institutional affiliations of all committee members are listed in the appendix. With substantial input from other participants in the first conference, the advisory committee members played a major role in defining the focus and setting the agenda for the meeting at which these papers were presented. We are indebted to them for this essential contribution.

Equally as important are the authors of the papers whose efforts make up the substance of the volume. Not only did they prepare and present these papers at the conference, but they responded conscientiously and good naturedly to the critiques, comments, and suggestions they received from conference participants through several rounds of review and revision. We are grateful to them all, as well as to those participants whose thoughtful and detailed commentaries helped to sharpen and refine the papers into the products that are published here. The list of participants in the conference is included in the appendix.

The contributions of the staff of the AAAS Directorate for Science and Policy Programs were also vital to the success of the conference and this book. Those involved include (in alphabetical order) Kamla Butaney, Magby Callejas, Audrey Chapman, Alexander Fowler, Elizabeth Gehman (formerly Broughman), Lauren Gelman (summer intern), and Deborah Runkle. We are indebted to them all. Cynthia Baskin, serving as a freelance editor, did an excellent and remarkably timely job of copyediting the manuscript and preparing it for publication. The staff of the AAAS Press, especially Louise Goines, provided encouragement, enthusiasm, and a congenial working relationship.

We are also most grateful to the Ethical, Legal, and Social Implications (ELSI) Program of the National Institutes of Health for supporting the project of which this conference and book are a part, and to its director, Eric Juengst, for his personal interest and involvement at all stages of the effort. The conference and this publication were also supported in part by the Department of Energy's ELSI program, through Los Alamos National Laboratory. We appreciate the support of this program, and especially the contributions and hospitality of its coordinator, Michael Yesley, who hosted the meeting at Los Alamos, and the assistance of Fran DiMarco of the Laboratory's Protocol Office, whose efforts helped to ensure a productive and enjoyable conference.

INTRODUCTION
Genetic Testing and the Human Genome Project

Albert H. Teich, Ph.D., and Mark S. Frankel, Ph.D.

The Human Genome Project and Its Implications

The inheritance of human traits—eye color, height, susceptibility to certain diseases—is, like the heredity of all organisms, shaped by units within cells known as genes. During the past several decades, researchers have unraveled the biochemical basis of genes. They have learned that genes are comprised of sequences of chemicals called nucleotides (or nucleotide bases) that link together to form long, complex molecules known as DNA. These DNA molecules pack together into the chromosomes that can be seen under a microscope in the nuclei of cells. There are four such nucleotides, and the order or sequence in which they are linked comprises a "code"—a means of preserving and transmitting information. It is this genetic code that contains the instructions that govern the structure and biochemical functions of the cells out of which all organisms are made. Taken together, an organism's complete set of genes—i.e., the totality of its genetic information—forms what is termed its "genome."

Recent developments in molecular biology have made it possible to identify specific sequences of DNA that are associated with individual traits of organisms. The Human Genome Project is an effort to decipher the complete genetic code of the human species. It involves both mapping (locating) all the genes in human DNA and sequencing (determining the order of nucleotides) for each of these genes. This is an immense task. It is estimated that the human genome contains between 50,000 and 100,000 genes and that they are encoded in as many as three billion pairs of nucleotides.

The Human Genome Project arose out of discussions among scientists in the mid 1980s who recognized the potential that new technologies of molecular biology and computers and information processing offered for understanding human development and genetic disorders. Begun in 1990, the project is expected to cost about $3 billion and take 15 years to complete. Funding (approximately $200 million per year) is being provided by the National Institutes of Health (NIH) and the U.S. Department of Energy. Related efforts are being conducted by scientists in a number of other countries. Unlike some "big science" projects, this project does not involve a single large device or laboratory on whose work rests the fate of the entire effort. Rather, the Genome Project is being conducted through the coordinated efforts of a large number of researchers in many different centers and laboratories. Its results, furthermore, are emerging piece by piece as the effort proceeds, and many of them—such as the identification of genes for colon cancer and cystic fibrosis—are already beginning to be applied in practice.

While the potential benefits of the Human Genome Project to society are enormous, there are also serious risks from the unanticipated consequences of this powerful new knowledge. The development of routine tests for predispositions to diseases and other human traits has profound implications for medical practice, for insurance, for the legal system, for employment practices, and for numerous other areas of society. Consider, for example, the prospect of being able to test a person at birth (or before) for susceptibility to several dozen genetically determined disorders, some of which may be treatable while others may not. How will the acquisition of this knowledge affect the social and economic status of this individual? His or her insurability or marriageability? What about the more remote prospect of being able to predict (and presumably choose) more complex traits such as athletic or musical ability, aspects of personality, or artistic talent? How will society deal with the issues that the emergence of such capabilities will raise? As a means of anticipating such risks and helping society reap the benefits of the new genetic knowledge while addressing in a constructive manner the potential dilemmas created by the products of the Human Genome Project, the designers of the project agreed to devote a portion of its resources to a program that has subsequently become known as the Ethical, Legal, and Social Implications (ELSI) Program. This book is a result of a two-year study by the American Association for the Advancement of Science (AAAS) supported by the ELSI Program.

The AAAS Genetic Testing Project

AAAS became involved in studying the ethical and legal implications of genetic testing through a convergence of interests of two of its constituent bodies—the Committee on Scientific Freedom and Responsibility (CSFR) and the National Conference of Lawyers and Scientists (NCLS). The CSFR was established in 1976 to, among other things, examine and consider responses to ethical issues associated with developments in science and technology. The NCLS is a joint venture of AAAS and the American Bar Association; its activities seek to explore issues at the intersection of science and law. Discussions that began independently in these two groups in the late 1980s led to the development of a collaborative project under which AAAS, in 1991 and 1992, convened a series of invitational conferences on ethical and legal implications of genetic testing. The project was intended to explore the most significant social concerns raised by advances in genetic technology and to help set a policy agenda to address these concerns. Invitees to the three conferences included scientists, ethicists, lawyers, health professionals, and representatives of interested parties (such as the pharmaceutical and insurance industries and genetic disease support groups).

The first of the three conferences, held in June 1991, provided an overview of ethical and legal issues raised by genetic testing in four areas of society: medical care and research, insurance, the workplace, and law enforcement and the courtroom. The meeting was intended to identify issues requiring further exploration and to eliminate others that were either beyond the reasonable scope of the project or being addressed satisfactorily by others (see American Association for the Advancement of Science 1992). Deliberations at the initial conference helped define the focus and set the agendas for the second and third meetings.

The second conference, held in March 1992, was devoted to ethical and legal aspects of pedigree research—i.e., genetic research that employs family trees, including tissue samples and medical data, to locate the genes for disorders or traits that are prevalent in these families (see American Association for the Advancement of Science, 1993). The third conference addressed a series of "frontier" ethical and legal issues raised by advances in genetic testing. These were issues of potentially broad and fundamental importance that could be created by the new technology of genetic testing and that might transcend sectors of society. Included on the agenda were the links between genetics, behavior, and responsibility; intellectual property and genetic testing; family relationships and social policy; and privacy and confidentiality. This conference was held in Los Alamos, New Mexico, in June 1992.

The Frontier Issues

The four topical areas that constitute the focus of this volume were chosen because they raise intriguing ethical and legal questions, as well as important policy issues. As much as any set of issues, they reflect the hopes, fears, prejudices, and uncertainties that people associate with the Human Genome Project. The essays presented here make no claim to allay those concerns, but they do attempt to provide an empirical base for deliberations on the issues, accompanied by an element of reasoned speculation.

As the chapters in Part I of this volume demonstrate, the family unit is in flux. Already redefined in the face of advancing reproductive technology and social pressures, family dynamics are likely to experience further changes as genetic testing becomes more prevalent and as our knowledge of human genetics grows. Whether these advances stabilize or erode the family unit and whether they illuminate or blur parental rights and duties remain to be determined.

Genetic testing will have a major impact on family planning and human reproduction as reliable tests to diagnose carrier and fetal genetic status increasingly become available. Decisions about whether to reproduce will raise difficult issues related to individual choice and social policy. Couples will have to wrestle responsibly with the nature of their obligations to reproduce, while society will need to consider whether social policy should attempt to influence individual choice. The excesses of past governmental efforts to intrude in reproductive decisions should properly caution us to view with apprehension any attempts at social intervention. Nevertheless, it is not unreasonable to question social policy that remains neutral in the face of what may be described as trivial or highly questionable parental preferences, such as progeny with blue eyes or sex selection.

The Human Genome Project, with its emphasis on genetic link-ages as the defining factor in human relationships, will also affect perceptions about the family. While genetic tests will reveal much about the biological ties among family members, families are more than individuals linked by similar DNA, and parenthood is determined and judged by more than genetics. One of the challenges ahead for social policy will be to make sensible use of the expanding knowledge about the influence of genetics on family health and functioning, while acknowledging the need to explore alternatives to the genetic model of the family.

The power and potential of genetics rest in the knowledge it provides, thereby raising concerns about privacy and confidentiality in a wide range of situations. The information gained from increased genetic knowledge will be of great interest to the affected individuals as well to others, including, for example, family members, employers, schools, insurers, and legal institutions. But such knowledge is a double-edged sword. On the one hand, knowledge of one's predisposition to a genetic disorder opens up the possibility of prevention or treatment. Even if nothing can be done to avoid the ill effects of the disorder, people will be able to make more informed decisions about their lives and their relationships with others.

On the other hand, the enhanced ability to identify genetic characteristics and genetic susceptibility to disease will undoubtedly affect the way people view themselves and how they are perceived by others. There is the possibility that some people who are informed of their genetic vulnerability, even if the risk is slight, will equate heredity with destiny and will believe that life offers them few real choices. And others, believing the same, may treat these people in a manner that restricts the way they live their lives, perhaps denying them access to social and economic opportunities. It is also possible that genetic knowledge will be used to classify people according to specific characteristics and capabilities that may subject them to new forms of discrimination, stigmatization, and control, either as individuals or as members of a particularly defined group.

Genetic information about an individual also can affect the privacy of other family members. Knowledge of a genetic condition that "runs in the family" raises concerns that other family members could be similarly vulnerable. This knowledge could influence important personal and family decisions regarding such matters as marriage, reproduction, and responsibility for the care of loved ones. In such situations, how does one balance the privacy rights of individuals and the confidentiality that have traditionally guided the patient—physician relationship with the competing health and social needs of other family members?

Efforts to establish DNA databanks for identification in law enforcement and the armed services also illustrate the conflict between an individual's preference for privacy and confidentiality and broader social needs. While accumulating evidence of criminal behavior and identifying the remains of military personnel are laudable social goals, the reality is that the possession of such DNA information by these bureaucratic institutions raises the specter of civil liberties violations that should concern all citizens. As the chapters in Part II readily demonstrate, society faces a series of challenging hurdles in deciding how to anticipate and respond to the generation and use of highly detailed information on the genetic makeup of individuals that will result from new technical capabilities produced by the Human Genome Project.

As illustrated by the chapters in Part III, behavioral genetics is the subject of some of the more contentious dialogue regarding the implications of the Human Genome Project. This is understandable in that research in behavioral genetics explores such matters as the nature of mental illness, antisocial behavior, and intelligence while attempting to account for the relative influence of heredity and environment on such characteristics. As we come closer to acquiring the ability to determine a person's genetic predisposition to certain types of behavior, we will be confronted by some very profound questions about what is meant by autonomy, responsibility, and culpability.

It is highly likely that most human behaviors are the result of some blend of genetic and environmental influences, but the nature of the mixture remains unresolved. Nevertheless, the remarkable success already attributed to the Human Genome Project in the medical arena may encourage some to embrace it as an explanatory framework for social problems as well. We must be alert to the danger of according too much authority to genetic knowledge. It is neither infallible nor determinative in many cases. In exploring its links to behavior, genetic knowledge should not routinely be allowed to trump other relevant factors, such as the environmental elements that influence the behavioral expression of a genetic condition.

While many people would embrace the notion of being unique individuals, they would just as readily avoid the label of being different. Genetics illuminates this paradox, as it seeks to identify, study, and explain differences among people as well as the uniqueness of individuals. As history has vividly demonstrated, emphasizing genetic differences, no matter how well grounded in science they may be, can have serious social and economic repercussions. This is especially true when genetics is used to highlight racial and ethnic differences.

The danger occurs when genetic differences are used to justify unequal treatment; to reinforce negative stereotypes that brand a group or person; or to ease our consciences about not undertaking efforts to reverse the social conditions that contribute to inequality or stigmatization. While racial and ethnic differences that affect health and disease must be acknowledged, we must be sensitive to potential abuse in light of the sordid history of the use of genetic information to support pernicious eugenic programs.

The topic of intellectual property examined in Part IV is especially timely, given the international debate precipitated by NIH's attempt to obtain patents on thousands of partial DNA sequences known as "expressed sequence tags," the functions or utility of which are unknown. The NIH contends that such patents are necessary so that the American biotechnology industry can be competitive in international markets. Many scientists, however, are outspoken in their criticism of those patenting efforts, based largely on their fear of an anticipated adverse impact on international cooperation and on the sharing of data. Although the NIH patent application was initially denied on legal and technical grounds, the more important question is whether seeking such protection constitutes wise social policy.

The underlying premise of intellectual property protection through patents is that advances in science will be promoted by granting exclusive rights for new discoveries, thereby offering an incentive to disclose those discoveries rather than keep them secret. In the past, such protection has served the interests of the pharmaceutical industry and the public by encouraging up-front investment in drug development with some assurance that companies would gain a profitable financial return on their initial investment.

In contemporary biotechnology research, the line between basic and applied research is becoming more and more blurred, fundamental knowledge has grown in economic importance, and researchers are increasingly involving themselves in commercial ventures. In this context, intellectual property protection is viewed by some as a threat to the generation and dissemination of knowledge by curbing scientific communication, by making it more difficult to gain access to the results of earlier research, and by creating the potential for prolonged litigation over patent results.

Science has traditionally operated under the principle of communal ownership of knowledge, where open communication and data sharing are perceived as essential for advancing science efficiently and cost effectively. This principle is reflected in the Human Genome Project, where large databases and repositories have been established to facilitate data sharing and to avoid duplication of effort and costly international competition. But the potential commercial value of genome research raises the question of how efforts to achieve an economic competitive advantage on the part of scientists, companies, or nations will affect the production and reporting of scientific research. Part IV of this volume examines the possible role that intellectual property protection will play in shaping the outcome of such efforts in the years ahead.

We hope this book will promote a heightened sensitivity to the new genetic frontier and will be helpful to the wide range of professionals engaged in genetics research and the assessment of its broader ethical, legal, and social implications, as well as to those individuals working through organized patient support groups to promote the use of genetics research in a manner that enhances health while preserving human dignity.

References

American Association for the Advancement of Science. 1992. *The Genome, Ethics and the Law: Issues in Genetic Testing.* AAAS Publication No. 92—115. Washington, DC: American Association for the Advancement of Science.

American Association for the Advancement of Science. 1993. *Ethical and Legal Issues in Pedigree Research.* Washington, DC: American Association for the Advancement of Science.

PART I

Family Relationships and
Social Policy

INTRODUCTION
Genes and Families

Robert Mullan Cook-Deegan, M.D.

The following chapters by Roger L. Shinn and R. Alta Charo give two different perspectives on how genetics may influence the changing nature of family relationships. Shinn offers an ethical and theological analysis of the historical alternatives to monogamous marriage and the impact of the sexual revolution on family relationships. Contemporary genetics is but one additional pressure on the traditional family, already reeling from changes in cultural norms, control of reproductive choice, and social factors that produce single-parent families, hybrid families from divorced and remarried parents, and gay marriages. With such a tumultuous shift, the degree and direction of change caused by advances in genetics are hard to predict.

If choosing a lifetime partner is a mix of romance and prudence—of irrational passion and rational assessment of compatibility—then new genetic knowledge will weigh in mainly on the side of prudence. More information about risks, both traits one's partner has or might develop and those that might appear in children of the union, may change family dynamics. Potential parents may choose not to have children, to avoid genetic risks through alternative reproductive methods such as artificial insemination, or to use genetic tests as a tool for deciding the characteristics of the children they will bear (Glover 1989, 1984). The consequences of these changes are again unpredictable, and they raise agonizing choices. Such opportunities were unavailable before the advent of genetic diagnostics, but with them come choices that never before had to be made. Barbara Katz Rothman has noted how in utero testing can perturb the course of a pregnancy, changing the experience for the woman, and often not for the better (Rothman 1987).

The new technological options present difficult social as well as individual choices. To what degree should policy attempt to influence individual choice? Shinn discusses the degree to which we will want to control our genetic destiny, both as individuals and collectively. This topic necessarily draws us into the shadow of eugenics and racial hygiene, inextricably mixed with the social history of genetics, and a topic of considerable contemporary scholarship (Kevles 1992, 1985; Wikler 1992; Adams 1990; Duster 1990; Gallagher 1990; Smith 1989; Müller-Hill 1988; Proctor 1988; Lifton 1986).

The central question now is the degree to which social goals should be allowed to influence decisions about who should be born and who should breed. The strong rejection of eugenics in the period since World War II is laudable, but taken to the extreme of nonintervention, it precludes action on some suspect practices. Should there be policies against sex selection, for example? Perspectives on this question differ around the world (Wertz and Fletcher 1989). A Working Group of the European Community that considered this question came to the conclusion, after considerable discussion, that governments should not intrude into *parental* choices but should discourage clinical services from proffering the service (Glover 1989). The force of government might work on institutions, but the fear of abuse was insufficient to warrant an assault on parental choices. To what degree should social policies be deliberately neutral about reproductive choices? Will parents be expected to bear the medical costs of a child knowingly born with a genetic disorder when prenatal testing was possible? There is much room for blaming parents and making them pay penalties for choices that fall outside social norms. The penalties could theoretically include financial burdens and social stigma.

If genetics becomes the basis for social judgments, it will do so through access to genetic information, raising the question of confidentiality. This topic is the subject of considerable discussion in other sections of this volume, but Shinn mentions it in the context of families. Shinn closes with a provocative observation. He speculates on whether we are living through a period of crosscurrents, with social forces yearning for "traditional family values" while also embracing technologies and cultural diversity that call into question whose traditions, whose family, and, most importantly, whose values.

R. Alta Charo reviews the way courts have used genetic rationales to justify disparate decisions. Adoption enabled individuals who were not genetically related to serve as parents. Artificial insemination by donors sundered the genetic connection between father and child. Courts struggled with ways to permit a "normal family" to persevere, while retaining a body of law intended to thwart women from cuckolding their husbands. Yet modern courts also employ genetics to link wayward fathers to their genetic children, under the theory that he who gets the pleasure should pay (a fair share of) the bills.

Courts, like society at large, tread an unmarked path through the new reproductive frontier. Surrogate motherhood, which Charo notes is itself rhetorically suspect and might better be termed "contract gestation," is not a genetic technology, but it does clearly demonstrate the three different kinds of parents: genetic, gestational, and postnatal or social. All three stages are equally "biological," but genetics has often been given more than its due. The confusing reality is dramatically illustrated by two Australian situations that mirror one another. In one case, a woman supplies the egg for an embryo implanted in her sister for gestation and rearing. In another case, a sister is the gestational mother for her sister's egg, and the child reverts to the genetic mother for rearing. In both cases, the altruistic sisters consider the mother to be the person who was intended all along to be the postnatal mother. The gestational mother giving the child to her sister declares she always felt like an aunt, while the sister who contributed an egg for her sister's gestation and birth feels the same way. These women clearly appreciate nuances that the courts are still struggling to grasp.

Charo argues for a strong presumption in favor of the gestational mother when custody of a child comes into dispute. The courts have occasionally shown a callous disregard for the health risks of pregnancy, the incredibly intimate and deep attachments that form during gestation, and the significant bodily risks of giving birth. When genetics trumps gestation, on the basis of who is the "biological" (erroneously taken to equate with genetic) mother, this ignores the much larger mass of biology beyond genetics; when intention to be the ultimate parent trumps the rights of a gestational mother, this signifies the triumph of contract over biology. The factors are complex and must be balanced, so a gestational mother cannot always carry the day, but the courts have in some cases had their thumbs on the scales of justice, casting aside the gestational mother who has taken the most personal risk and made the greatest psychological investment in a pregnancy.

Charo also exhorts us to open our laws to embrace the complexities of relationships. A child can have many parents of different kinds. She notes the desires of gay couples to raise children and the contradictions raised by attempting to force every family to resemble the "two parent (mother and father)-with-children" model. The legal argument here is that courts have been inconsistent, and this inconsistency traces ultimately to largely uninspected notions of family norms. Cannot there be a different kind of family, with many people having different kinds of relationships to a child? The answer may be yes, but getting there is not a straight shot.

Given the inconsistencies in the law, it seems likely that courts have been right at times and wrong at other times. The problem with purely legal analysis is that it does not, and cannot, set a gold standard when the criteria for deciding what is right or wrong are part of what is at stake. Should courts permit gay couples to adopt? Should they ensure that single women can have artificial insemination? If the best interests of children are taken as the primary goal, then the legal precepts should follow some analysis of what those interests are. But where are the data? Charo implicitly accepts the benefits of the diverse child-rearing practices she foresees, and there are plausible arguments that children may be better off with legally sanctioned relationships to more than a single mother-father couple (by whatever definition one wishes to choose). Guidance on children's best interests, however, depends not on legal analysis but on a reliable body of empirical data about how children fare under alternative family arrangements and how the specific child whose life is being considered by a court will fare. The legal arguments for a more flexible and permissive interpretation of family structure would carry a great deal more weight if based on actual data about children's experiences. Here, legal arguments reach a limit that can only be surmounted when the social and biological sciences provide some answers.

Courts are generally brought in to settle disputes. It is in just such situations that the value of multitudinous attachments may be most questionable. A judge trying to decide a case must often choose who shall have custody over a child. An important part of the judge's decision is determining who will decide for the child. An impassioned battle between husband and wife is difficult enough to resolve. Bringing in the egg donor, sperm donor, gestational mother, and perhaps others with legitimate claims of attachment further complicates the decision. In physics, the two-body problem can theoretically be solved, although sometimes after considerable contortion; but the many-body problem has no general solution. Judges may be forgiven for relying on tradition when it may be the only guide, and they are certain to endure strident criticism for departing from it. Asking the courts to open themselves to alternative family arrangements amid familial strife, in just those situations where the alternative structure has bred conflict, may be less promising than asking the social sciences to produce evidence that the new structures produce healthy and happy children. Then the courts can decide based on evidence.

These twin chapters blaze two trails into the genetic frontier, one following theological and ethical analysis and the other legal analysis of how genetic information is used in family law. Both point to the increasingly obvious fact that progress in one science, genetics, is exposing the need for inquiry in psychology, sociology, anthropology, economics, and other social sciences. We talk much about families—theology and the law embody our musings—but we know relatively little about what happens when we alter their structure. Families will increasingly confront choices brought about by advances in genetic tests and general knowledge about genetics. The scientific exploration of the genetic frontier invites, nay necessitates, exploration of frontiers in the social sciences.

References

Adams, M.B., ed. 1990. *The Wellborn Science: Eugenics in Germany, France, Brazil, and Russia.* New York: Oxford University Press.

Duster, T. 1990. *Backdoor to Eugenics.* New York: Routledge.

Gallagher, H.G. 1990. *By Trust Betrayed: Patients and Physicians in the Third Reich.* New York: Henry Holt.

Glover, J. 1989. *Fertility and the Family: The Glover Report on New Reproductive Technologies.* The European Commission. London: Fourth Estate.

Glover, J. 1984. *What Sort of People Should There Be?* London: Penguin, Harmondsworth.

Kevles, D.J. 1992. "Out of Eugenics: The Historical Politics of the Human Genome." In D.J. Kevles and L. Hood, eds., *The Code of Codes: Scientific and Social Issues in the Human Genome Project.* Cambridge: Harvard University Press.

Kevles, D.J. 1985. *In the Name of Eugenics.* Berkeley: University of California Press.

Lifton, R.J. 1986. *The Nazi Doctors.* New York: Basic Books.

Müller-Hill, B. 1988. *Murderous Science.* New York: Oxford University Press.

Proctor, R.N. 1988. *Racial Hygiene: Medicine Under the Nazis.* Cambridge: Harvard University Press.

Rothman, B.K. 1987. *The Tentative Pregnancy: Prenatal Diagnosis and the Future of Motherhood.* New York: Penguin Books.

Smith, J.D. and Nelson, K.R. 1989. *The Sterilization of Carrie Buck.* Far Hills, NJ: New Horizon Press.

Wertz, D.C. and Fletcher, J.C. 1989. *Ethics and Human Genetics: A Cross-Cultural Perspective.* New York: Springer-Verlag.

Wikler, D. and Palmer, E. 1992. "Neo-Eugenics and Disability Rights in Philosophical Perspective." In N. Fujiki and D.R.J. Macer, eds., *Human Genome Research and Society: Proceedings of the Second International Bioethics Seminar in Fukui, 20–21 March, 1992* 105–113. Christchurch, NZ: Eubios Ethics Institute.

1

Family Relationships and Social Policy: An Ethical Inquiry

Roger L. Shinn, Ph.D.

For aeons of history, genetic beliefs have been a mix of folklore, superstition, prejudice (tribal, racial, class, national, imperial), hunches, and uncritical generalizations. There are traces of genetic theory, error-ridden and often vicious, in myths of many cultures, in epics of East and West, and in scriptures of several religions. High philosophies did little better: Plato and Aristotle engaged in genetic speculations and recommendations, now easily recognized as nonsense.

However, since the mid-nineteenth century, elements of a genuine genetic science have emerged, recently with dazzling speed. The uncertainties are still immense. Specialists argue endlessly over the difference between "nature and nurture." Proposals to study the relation between genetics and crime lead to loud protests, rising out of fear that the investigation will be motivated by, or the results appropriated by, pernicious ideologues. Even so, a burst of scientific activity has produced a mass of verifiable information, along with the power to diagnose and treat serious diseases. Yet the new knowledge and power may be frightening in their potentialities.

The family is far older than genetic theory, but it has taken many structures throughout history. A fantasist might imagine some forms of family life that have not been tried, but that would take some doing. Amid all the varieties, it may be possible to discern a general trend, with numerous exceptions, toward the monogamous family. In its idealized form, children are born of a marriage and grow up with a mother and a father. The many exceptions include polygamy (usually polygyny, more rarely polyandry), concubinage, exploitation of slaves, group marriages, and unintended births from fleeting sexual relations. But on most continents there has been a widespread recognition of an ideal: children are born of a voluntary—mutually voluntary—sexual union of a man and a woman, who live in a continuing relationship of responsibility toward each other and toward the children.

It has become a cliché to say that the nuclear family of Norman Rockwell's America is a culture-specific type. But the monogamous family became, not only in middle America, a cultural norm, often violated but generally acknowledged, supported by social practice and law. A test case in the United States was Mormon polygamy (polygyny), which led to a congressional act against polygamy in 1862 and a Supreme Court decision upholding the law in 1879.(1)

Monogamy, ideally and often in practice, restrained predatory sexuality and indiscriminate paternity by males. *Men* had a stake in monogamy: Since maternity is an undeniable event while paternity can be denied, monogamy gave men some assurance that children were biologically their own. That concern could be maintained in polygyny, but by considerable effort and expense—to take an extreme example, the maintenance of a harem supervised by eunuchs. *Women* had a stake in monogamy: It gave mothers some security during pregnancy and in continuing family relations. Margaret Mead (1955, ch. IX), in a chapter title, declared: "Fatherhood [unlike motherhood] Is a Social Invention."(2) She saw such inventions as "infinitely fragile," requiring constant nurture. *Children* also had a stake in monogamy: It provided them with two parents in a presumably stable home and, to use an overworked term, both male and female role models.

Abuses of monogamy were frequent. Many societies assumed a double standard of morality, asking of women a sexual discipline that males did not practice. Present American society recognizes how patriarchal its traditional family was. Too often men considered women and children to be legal property rather than sharers in an intimate and responsible relationship. So the authority of traditional norms is increasingly challenged.

Simultaneously, economic changes are revising past assumptions that women are normally economic dependents. The increasing economic capability of women is one reason why family unions are, for better or worse, less permanent than in the past, particularly in industrial societies.

These cultural changes, proceeding in many societies, have been accelerated by developments in biological and medical science that open up new options. Sexual activity without reproduction has become easy—although not so easy as to avoid many unintended pregnancies. Even more innovative is the practice of reproduction without sexual intercourse. Artificial insemination, whether by husband (AIH) or by donor (AID), makes conception a clinical process. In vitro fertilization goes still further in separating conception from sexual intimacy. The press reports that "the business of high-tech baby making is booming," with more than

$1 billion spent on fertility services in 1992 (Miller et al. 1992, 38). While these processes are sometimes welcomed by husband and wife, they are technologically just as available outside the relationship of marriage. The combination of cultural, biological, and technological developments means an increase in single parents, usually female but sometimes male. The current estimate is that, of eight million single-parent families in the United States, about 15 percent or 1.2 million are headed by males (of whom only 7.5 percent are widowers) (Seligman 1992, 70). Some lesbian couples are parents, with one of the two a biological mother. Gay couples have become parents, usually by adoption.

These changes, so fast and extensive, stir furious controversies. People ask which of our social ills are related to the instability of the family. No-fault divorce, introduced as an enlightened arrangement, especially as compared with the acrimony of past proceedings, has proved economically hard on women and children. It is reported that in the United States, almost half the families headed by a single woman, whether unmarried or divorced, live below the poverty line.(3) The paradox is that the economic—cultural changes that enhance opportunities for some women intensify poverty for others—and their children.

Public debates rage over the relationships between sexual permissiveness and the surge of teenage parents, high infant mortality, unemployment, homelessness, crime, drug traffic, and the spread of Autoimmune Deficiency Syndrome (AIDS). An international medical study, headed by Dr. Myrna Weissman, finds a major increase in depression over the past three decades, especially among youth (even allowing for improved reporting of the phenomenon) (Cross-National 1992).(4) Dr. Frederick Goodwin, director of the National Institute of Mental Health, which was one of the sponsors of the research, sees a principal cause as the "tremendous erosion of the nuclear family" and the virtual disappearance of the extended family (Goleman 1992). On issues like this, nobody can trace cause and effect with precision. The uncertainty of the issues invites simplified answers and political exploitation. In the public mind, "liberal" politics has been related to permissiveness, the breakdown of traditional disciplines, and decline of the family. "Conservative" politics has embraced traditional family values. But on the far right the libertarians have upset those linkages, and on the moderate left the recent "communitarian" movement has joined "liberal" economic policies with an appreciation of traditional values. In the political campaign of 1992, the polemics became both demagogic and comic, as politicians and fictional television personalities joined in.

Most of this has taken place independently of the new genetic knowledge. But genetic science, both in the clinic and in popular culture, interacts with these other developments. It is the interaction that is so potent with alluring, yet perilous possibilities.

Some Specific Issues

Genetic Testing of Parents or Prospective Parents

Genetic testing, quite impossible to earlier generations, is now widely practiced. Suppose family histories give some reason to suspect that two married persons, apparently healthy, carry the gene for an ailment that can be discovered by testing.

That situation, although fairly simple, already includes one problematic word—ailment. We could use a stronger word, disease, or a weaker one, anomaly; but the issue remains. Normality is not a purely biological concept; it is also cultural. To take an obvious example, skin color has often been a liability—economically, legally, educationally, residentially, and professionally. Such liabilities result in medical liabilities—high infant mortality, high victimization by violence, and a lower life expectancy associated with high blood pressure. But there is no biological or ontological inevitability in these associated liabilities. Society imposes them. The answer is not a medical or genetic program to modify skin color. When society learns that black (or brown or red or yellow) is beautiful, the liability disappears.

Even so, there are some genetically transmitted qualities that nobody could wish for self or offspring—deficiencies that bring great pain, disintegration of physical and mental capacity, and early death. No responsible parent, in any social situation, could wish these deficiencies on children. I use the term "ailment" for such liabilities.

The example most often used is Tay-Sachs disease. I use this example with some trepidation, again for social reasons. It is most frequent among Ashkenazi Jews, emerging in one out of about every thirty-six hundred births. That fact can be used to feed prejudice or support arguments of ethnic inferiority. The simple answer is that other people are more vulnerable to other ailments; for example, people of North European descent are more liable to cystic fibrosis, the most common genetic ailment in the United States, affecting one in about every eighteen hundred white people (Lee 1991).(5) I use the example of Tay-Sachs because it is more susceptible than most ailments to genetic testing and prediction.

The recessive trait leads to no symptoms. But if both parents carry the gene, then the probability of the disease, in the familiar Mendelian pattern, is one out of four for each of their children. A man and a woman, wanting to marry, frequently ask for genetic testing. If they discover that their offspring will be at risk, they face several options. They can decide not to marry and, perhaps with painful realization, seek other marital partners. They can decide to marry and not procreate: to maintain a childless marriage, to adopt a child, to seek pregnancy through AID—after the donor, of course, has been tested for this liability. (The donor, like the marital couple, cannot be tested for all liabilities; there is no pregnancy without genetic risk.) They can procreate, accepting the risk. Or they can go ahead with a pregnancy, arranging a prenatal testing of the fetus, with abortion as a possibility.

This procedure, as it becomes available for more ailments, may become typical of "the brave new world" that humanity is entering. It raises a host of ethical issues with political and social dimensions. Will families be blamed for passing on genetic liabilities that they could have prevented? Will government and insurance companies pick up the bills for expensive treatments that might have been prevented? Should genetic testing—of parents for recessive traits or of fetuses—ever be mandated, regardless of the wishes of parents?

We can already begin to see some changes in practices of courtship and marriage. Sexual attraction is a combination of the impulsive and unpredictable with the calculable and prudent. The man and woman directly involved may not bother to analyze the nature of this combination, but history and literature have already done that.

The tradition of romantic love, celebrated in legend and poetry and fiction, takes its extreme form in the reckless passion that is indifferent to consequences. Prudent obstacles make it all the more alluring. Denis de Rougement (1956) has traced the history of romantic love, with the story of Tristan and Iseult as his prime example.

Prudent marriage has its strongest expression in the practice of arranged marriages. The most common form involves parental agreement, sometimes prolonged bargaining, quite indifferent to the personal choices of the children or youths who are destined to marry. It takes place today in the mass marriages or "Blessings" of the Unification Church, where marital partners are designated by the Reverend Sun Myung Moon. Our society, with its ethos of individualism, tends to scorn the idea of arranged marriages, but there is more of the prudent element in marriage than popular culture acknowledges. Despite exceptions, people tend to marry within their social class, not with the rigidity of, say, the Hindu caste system, but with what biologists and sociologists call "assortative mating."

What happens is usually something like this: I (or some other I) find so-and-so attractive. I do not immediately think about whether I would like so-and-so to be the parent of my children. But sooner or later I may entertain that question, along with a lot of other prudent interests, especially economic. These interests have already been operating subconsciously from the first attraction.

The increase of genetic testing will probably heighten the prudent element in marriage. (There is some evidence that fear of AIDS has done so in casual sexual encounters.) One can imagine new caution about hidden liabilities. How far this will go, I cannot guess. It would, for example, be hard to imagine a rewriting of *Romeo and Juliet* to include a scene for genetic testing. It would be equally hard to revise the popular song of my childhood to run: "The blue of her eyes and the gold of her hair/and the health of her DNA." But Romeo and Juliet and the "Sweetheart of Sigma Chi" are not popular paradigms for the family patterns of the future.

Herman Muller's Proposals

For a second example, I turn to the proposals some years ago of Herman Muller, a geneticist and Nobel laureate in biology. His ideas were quite independent of genetic testing, but they are applicable to a world where genetic testing has become more frequent than in his time. They form a test case for decisions on how far we want to separate procreation from the traditional family relationship.

Muller was an enthusiast for eugenics—the effort to improve the genetic heritage of the human race on a large scale. He thought—as recently as 1967—that genetic engineering (genetic surgery, as he called it) would never be possible. He could then not guess that enzymes (chemical scissors) would do what scalpels could never do. He thus advocated a massive use of sperm banks for AID.(6)

Muller urged that the sperm of distinguished men be used for artificial insemination. He hoped that many men would generously yield their traditional prerogatives to superior genetic fathers. The proposal would not change the structure of the family or the quality of sexual intimacy, except that sexual union would be radically dissociated from procreation. One would take place at home, the other in a hospital or doctor's office.

Muller acknowledged difficulties in picking genetic fathers. Looking at the past, he proposed Darwin as an ideal progenitor. Lenin was a conspicuous name on an early list, conspicuously absent later. Muller was, in fact, deeply pessimistic that so degenerate a society as ours would choose wisely. For that reason, he suggested that frozen sperm be preserved for 20 years before use, to allow a sound judgment on the worth of genetic fathers. Muller's successors were less patient. In 1977 they set up a sperm bank in California, securing donations from five Nobel laureates in science, who could be presumed to confer an ideal heredity on future children (Schmeck, Jr. 1980, 60). Although they named it for Muller, they were far less ambitious than he. Initially, at least, they released sperm only for impregnation of married women unable to have children by their husbands, a limitation that would have been a disappointment to Muller. They further required permission of the husband.

These restraints are clearly not based on genetic science. They are social and ethical, whether because of the beliefs of the sponsors of the sperm bank or because of deference to public opinion. There is no scientific reason why sperm from the bank could not be made available to single women, lesbian partners, or to wives unwilling to inform husbands.

Since Muller, in vitro fertilization has made possible an expansion of his idea. Both genetic parents, not just the father, can be selected for genetic reasons. Thus far, banks of frozen ova have not proved practical, but that may change. This prospect has led to speculations about "genetic supermarkets," where parents might shop for the sperm and ova that would give their children a superior heredity.

Critics have accused Muller of naiveté about the relation between genetics and personality—about the relation between heredity, environment, and human freedom (see the chapters by Anderson and Cole-Turner in this book). But a more modest application of his ideas might be the use of sperm banks when genetic testing shows liabilities in prospective parents. The broader use, which he advocated, requires individuals and society to ask how much they value the "natural" linkage of reproduction with the intimate sexual relationship.

As to the effect of such proposals on family life, we can only conjecture. Henry Ford, when he pioneered mass production of automobiles, did not know what he was doing to habits of dating, sexual relationships, and family life. Nor did anybody else. We are about as ignorant on the outcomes for the family of new genetic techniques. But we can be more alert to the issues.

Genetic Therapy

With genetic therapy we come to a very different possibility. It may become feasible to let the old-fashioned process of procreation go ahead, with confidence that the genetic ailment can be healed. Nobody should assume that humanity is on the verge of a utopia of good health. The best early possibilities—far from certainties—are for the correction of a very few identifiable ailments. With new discoveries the list will presumably expand. But there is no reason to expect refutation of the insight, imbedded deeply in the folk wisdom of many cultures and religions, that human life is inherently frail and vulnerable.

Proposed gene therapies take two forms. The more modest is the transplantation of genes into somatic cells, freeing the individual from a specific liability. This form of therapy entered the testing phase in 1990. In 1992, experimenters at Case Western Reserve University removed cells of a brain tumor from rats, altered the cells genetically, reinjected them into the rats, and found that the tumors regressed (Trojan et al. 1993).

At about the same time, the National Institutes of Health permitted physicians to inject a woman with her own genetically altered cells in the hope of curing a brain tumor (Associated Press 1992).(7) It is too early to make confident predictions about the future of such techniques.

The second, more radical form of gene therapy proposes a comparable treatment of human germ cells, extending the benefits to future generations. One outcome of the current Human Genome Initiative may be a contribution to such therapy. But the processes are extremely intricate. They may produce disastrous and irreparable side effects persisting into future generations. Some eminent scientists oppose the adventure. The late Erwin Chargaff of Columbia University, who discovered the base complementarity in nucleic acids, issued the challenge (1978, 190): "Have we the right to counteract, irreversibly, the evolutionary wisdom of millions of years, in order to satisfy the ambition and the curiosity of a few scientists?"(8) That language may express Chargaff's personal irascibility, as he wryly acknowledged. But more recently the Council for Responsible Genetics (1992) issued a position paper that, on "scientific, ethical, and social" grounds, "strongly opposes the use of germ line gene modification in humans."(9)

Federal guidelines at present forbid the altering of germline cells. But that prohibition may be temporary. It is far different from an accepted principle that genetic and medical science should never modify germline cells in the interest of therapy. Two ecumenical church groups, while emphasizing the gravity of any attempts to modify human germplasm, carefully avoided calling for a permanent prohibition. The National Council of the Churches of Christ in the U.S.A. (1986, 4, 13) adopted a policy statement in 1986, warning against the dangers of genetic manipulation and urging "extreme caution" and "especially stringent control" if germline therapy should ever become practical. The World Council of Churches (1989, 2), through its Central Committee, proposed "a ban on experiments involving genetic engineering of the human germline at the present time" and encouraged "the ethical reflection necessary for developing future guidelines in this area."(10)

The Commission for the Study of Ethical Problems in Medicine and Biomedical and Behavioral Research (1982, 56), appointed by former President Carter, called for "especially stringent" precautions but concluded: "To turn away from gene splicing, which may provide a means of curing hereditary diseases, would itself raise serious ethical problems."

Future developments will depend on the interaction between scientific research and the formation of public policy. Defining the "future guidelines" and the "especially stringent" precautions remains a foreboding task, which will be addressed later in this chapter.

Issues of Privacy

Genetic testing discloses information about an individual that would otherwise remain unknown. According to the prevailing ethic of the physician—patient relationship, much of that information remains confidential. But in the case of DNA "fingerprinting," some information (discoverable from a hair or some blood or sperm left at the scene of a crime) may be no more confidential than a fingerprint that identifies a thief.

The first is the question of disputes about rape and paternity. Genetic fingerprinting offers possibilities of more accurate identification of the males involved. Such tests can establish both accountability and innocence. When a conviction of an accused rapist was overturned in the Suffolk (NY) County Court in 1992, the defense attorneys stated that, in at least a dozen cases in the past two years, DNA tests had exonerated the defendant (Rabinovitz 1992). (In other cases, the tests have vindicated the accuser.) Continuing questions about the adequacy of the method used by testing laboratories involve scientific judgments. If they are clarified, the testing accords with established ethical practices of our society.

The more perplexing issue arises in the case of confidentiality. Suppose genetic tests discover a severe liability in a married man. Usually he wants to tell his wife. But suppose he does not. Does the physician have any responsibility to inform the wife in cases where the liability may impose a severe burden on her? Ray White, a pioneer in developing techniques for mapping the human genome, has asked (Bishop and Waldholz 1991, 270), "Will there be a statutory requirement for a man and woman to share genetic information before they marry and could failure to disclose genotype become grounds for divorce?" Others have suggested that "obstetricians might be liable to malpractice suits if they didn't test prospective couples who later conceived a child" affected by Tay-Sachs disease (Bishop and Waldholz 1991, 190).

A comparable question arose on the issue of AIDS at a conference in New York (Conference 1967). Some lawyers judged that the patient might sue the doctor if the doctor broke confidentiality and informed the wife. But the wife, if she acquired AIDS, might sue the doctor for failing to warn her, especially if the wife is also a patient of the doctor. Does the doctor have a responsibility to inform other women whom he knows to be sexually involved with the man (1) if they are his patients or (2) if they are not? Since AIDS is an infectious disease and genetic ailments are not infectious, does genetic information have a higher claim to confidence? On such technicalities many a legal case hangs. Can ethics pay such attention to technicalities? Can it avoid them? Here, as so often in medical ethics, scientific advances push persons and societies onto unmapped ethical terrain.

The subject of ethics has been discussed thus far by highlighting various beliefs about family, marriage, monogamy, and reproduction. Even allowing for diversity within and among populations, individuals and societies do have ethical beliefs, some of which have been codified in law. Given the real and potential discoveries in genetic science, the question remains: How do individuals, families, subcultures, cultures, and governments develop a prescriptive ethic, one that establishes rules, a direction, an order?

Our society is currently in the midst of great confusion and change. It is exhibiting and experiencing two opposing trends of thought and of action. One movement is the relaxation or rejection of some traditional ethical restraints. Old legalisms look quaint, inappropriate, even pernicious. The equally obvious countercurrent is an increasing ethical stringency on some issues: the wrongs of racism, ecological destructiveness, gender discrimination, and sexual harassment. Laws, regulations, and corporate policies forbid behavior that was ignored or even accepted a generation ago.

These counter tendencies—toward moral relaxation or moral rigor—do not always conflict with one another. Sound reasons can and do exist for rejecting some old prescriptions and enforcing new rules. However, on a number of controversial issues having highly emotional and widely divergent viewpoints, individuals and society are still struggling to define, express, and codify their beliefs. Arguments continue to rage, most obviously on the topics of reproductive ethics and abortion. The public is uneasy about genetics, aware of the vicious history of past eugenic movements, suspicious of manipulation, yet hopeful about relief from devastating diseases. At this point in human history, society is facing the challenge of making unprecedented decisions, prompted by new scientific knowledge and technological power.

Andrew Delbanco (1992, 41) of Columbia University has defined "the leading intellectual problem of our time: the effort to move from the skeptical to the constructive mood; to come to terms with the discovery that rationality is just one in the infinite range of possible cultural performances; to remake a human world at a time when the human 'sciences' seem devoted to exposing their own arbitrariness." What is the basis of ethics, particularly in a time of diverse values and angry disagreements? History shows two frequent, typical attempts to escape the slippery slope to nihilism. The first is to establish an unchallengeable ethical authority—rational, political, or religious. Plato tried, with his realm of pure ideas. Kant tried, with an irrefutable practical reason. Governments have tried, with the imposed will of a dictator or a popular majority. Religious communities have tried, with a sacred scripture or a priesthood. Always there have been dissenters, and many of them have prevailed over time.

The second attempt has been to make ethics a science, subject to verification by empirical methods. The ancient Epicureans sought to root ethics in a reckoning of pleasure and pain, as though these were self-evident criteria. Modern utilitarianism added a more sophisticated calculation of consequences. But the estimate of consequences leads at best to probabilities, and any understanding of human behavior shows that pleasure is not an unquestionable good and pain is not an absolute evil—unless one defines these terms in complex ways that reinstate all the old arguments that utilitarianism had hoped to resolve.

The valid insight of utilitarianism is its recognition that there is an element of calculation in all ethics except possibly the most formal and abstract. Any decisions about actual policy require empirical information and an estimate (never quite certain) of situations and consequences. They require also a weighing of various values. We want reduced crime without intolerable regimentation and coercion. We want the double sexual freedom: freedom for sexual expression and freedom from unwanted attention. We want a human society with less of a genetic load, provided we can get it without unacceptable hazards or infringement on personal freedom. In all these cases, social policy must consult the sciences—obviously the behavioral sciences but, especially in the case of genetics, the natural sciences as well. I suspect that the sciences will play an increasing role in the ethics of the future. An example of this, which has already been mentioned, is found in the devising of guidelines for possible genetic therapies.

This is not to call for a new scientific priesthood, prescribing conduct like the more sacerdotal priesthoods of the past. Werner Heisenberg (1960, 230) was surely right in finding it "impossible to base articles of belief that are to be binding for one's bearing in life on scientific knowledge alone."

Alfred North Whitehead (1925, 11) wrote: "Every philosophy is tinged with the colouring of some secretive imaginative background, which never emerges explicitly into its trains of reasoning." That is nowhere more evident than in the various human meanings of the family. As Kathryn Allen Rabuzzi (1987, 276) has observed, "Historically and cross-culturally, family in various forms has (until the late twentieth century in postindustrialized cultures) been so basic to human existence as to be a universal symbol of ultimacy." The symbolisms have been fantastically diverse. They have legitimated cruelty as well as compassion. Neither Zeus nor Shiva is a healthy role model for husbands and fathers. Yet we must ask whether the absence of all symbols of ultimacy means emptiness or even nihilism.

The "secret imaginative background," especially when it comes to ethics, refers to what it is to be human, to live in responsible relations to others, to posterity, and to the natural and cosmic sources of life. It is often embedded in myth. Throughout most of human history it has usually been related to religion. Today it may be that the most influential mythmakers of our society exercise their powers less in formal religion than in enterprises in Hollywood, on Wall Street and Madison Avenue, and inside the Washington beltway.

Max Weber (1958, 117) argued that science can contribute much to ethics by discovering new knowledge and showing how means relate to ends. But the choice of ends, he said, is finally "a matter of faith." Even in politics, perhaps most certainly in politics, "some kind of faith must always exist." Some of us still find powerful resources in traditional faiths. But faiths, conspicuously in our present world, differ. The secular and humanistic religions of our time also differ in their judgments as to how far a public ethic should prescribe and legally codify standards of conduct, as evident in debates on equality (especially concerning race and gender), affirmative action, and a host of comparable issues. Public policy must take account of those differences.

The great ethical traditions, whether religious or philosophical, developed largely before modern science, particularly genetic science, which requires decisions that past generations never faced. That puts an ethical responsibility on the scientific community—to inform the public (now very ill-informed about genetic developments), to alert the society to new hopes and perils, and to participate like other citizens in the shaping of policy. The least powerful in society have as much at stake in genetics as the most brilliant scientists but cannot make sound judgments without scientific information and insights.

There are some signs that today's multicultural world may be moving toward something like a consensus, shaky but persistent, on issues of human dignity, rights, and responsibilities. The United Nations Universal Declaration of Human Rights may be a sign. It is often violated, but even tyrants are slow to deny it publicly. Something of this sensitivity may give a basis for a multicultural ethic that is more than an aimless floundering. It may contribute to a search that will draw on treasured traditions even as it innovates, a search that welcomes the insights of science while it acknowledges the mystery of selfhood and responsibility.

There is hope that the search will confirm some traditional values of fidelity, stability, and responsibility in the family and that it will refuse to reduce the person to a mechanism of replaceable parts. Perhaps it will enhance human powers of healing. It may, by removing some fears that were the sanctions of past moral prohibitions, help people discover what they really want in the relations of sexuality and family. Beyond that, it is impossible to predict or prescribe.

Four decades ago Bertrand Russell wrote (1953, 97—98): "The human race has survived hitherto owing to ignorance and incompetence; but, given knowledge and competence combined with folly, there can be no certainty of survival. Knowledge is power, but it is power for evil just as much as for good. It follows that, unless men increase in wisdom as much as in knowledge, increase of knowledge will be an increase of sorrow." To the perilous leaps in power, associated with war and ecology, we must now add genetic knowledge. Past genetic theories, usually infected with prejudice, have brought the world much sorrow. An ethical imagination, this time around, might do better. The historical record gives us no assurance of that heightened insight, but it allows us to hope.

Notes

1. President James Buchanan removed Mormon Brigham Young from the governorship of the territory of Utah in 1857, then sent troops to quell the protests. Congress acted against polygamy in 1862, and the Supreme Court upheld the act in 1879. In 1890 the church dropped its authorization of polygamy, thus making it politically feasible for Utah to attain statehood in 1890. One wonders whether the congressional act or decision of the Supreme Court would be likely today (Ahlstrom 1972, 501–509, esp. 507).

2. The book was first published in 1949. Six years later in the edition quoted here, Mead (1955, vi–viii) added the statement: "For, while it still may be said that there seems to be no instinctive basis for fatherhood as such in human beings, evidence is mounting for the probability that the human male shares with non-human males, mammals and birds both, a protective response to the very young of his own species."

3. Marriott (1992, 1) attributes the data to a report of the Ways and Means Committee of the House of Representatives.

4. The study took place in nine countries: the United States, Canada, Puerto Rico, Germany, Italy, France, Lebanon, New Zealand, and Taiwan.

5. See Lee (1991), p. 263, on Tay-Sachs disease, p. 188, on cystic fibrosis.

6. Muller's ideas were expressed in various writings over a period of time. This section is primarily drawn from his final formulation, "What Genetic Course Will Man Steer?," in Crow and Neel (1967).

7. The procedure is here described as the "first" attempt to "to use an unproven gene therapy on a woman dying from a brain tumor."

8. Chargaff is reproducing his letter to the editor here, first published in *Science* 192:938–940 (June 4, 1976).

9. The CRG describes itself as "a Cambridge [MA]-based national organization of scientists, public health advocates, trade unionists, women's health activists and others who want to see biotechnology developed safely and in the public interest." It includes several prominent biological scientists.

10. I participated in studies of both groups that led to these formal actions but had no hand in the final formulations quoted here.

References

Ahlstrom, S. 1972. *A Religious History of the American People*. New Haven, CT: Yale University Press.

Associated Press. 1992. "Patient to Get Gene Therapy." *New York Times* (December 30) A12.

Bishop, J.E. and Waldholz, M. 1991. *Genome*. Touchstone ed. New York: Simon and Schuster.

Chargaff, E. 1978. *Heraclitean Fire: Sketches from a Life Before Nature*. New York: Rockefeller University Press.

Commission for the Study of Ethical Problems in Medicine and Biomedical and Behavioral Research. 1982. *Splicing Life: The Social and Ethical Issues of Genetic Engineering with Human Beings*. Washington, DC: U.S. Government Printing Office.

Conference on "AIDS: Humanistic Perspectives." February 26–27, 1967. Sponsored by the Department of Epidemiology and Social Medicine, Montefiore Medical Center/Albert Einstein College of Medicine, supported by The New York Council for the Humanities and other sources, at The New School for Social Research, New York.

Council for Responsible Genetics (CRG). 1992, Fall. "Position Paper on Human Germ Line Manipulation."

Cross-National Collaborative Group. 1992. "The Changing Rate of Major Depression." *Journal of the American Medical Association (JAMA)* 268: 3098–3105.

Crow, J.F. and Neel, J.V., eds. 1967. *Proceedings of the Third International Conference of Human Genetics*. Baltimore: Johns Hopkins University Press.

Delbanco, A. 1992. "The Skeptical Pilgrim." *New Republic* (July 6) 41.

de Rougement, D. 1956. *Love in the Western World* rev. augmented ed. New York: Pantheon Books Inc.

Goleman, G. 1992. "A Rising Cost of Modernity: Depression." *New York Times* (December 8) C13.

Heisenberg, W. 1960. "The Representation of Nature in Contemporary Physics." In R. May, ed., *Symbolism in Religion and Literature*. New York: George Braziller.

Lee, T.F. 1991. *The Human Genome Project: Cracking the Genetic Code of Life*. New York: Plenum Press.

Marriott, M. 1992. "Fathers Find That Child Support Means Owing More than Money." *New York Times* (July 20) 1.

Mead, M. 1955. *Male and Female: A Study of the Sexes in a Changing World*. New York: The New American Library of World Literature.

Miller, A., Friday, C., and King, P. 1992. "Baby Makers Inc." *Newsweek* (June 29) 38.

Murray, T.H. 1992. "The Human Genome Project and Genetic Testng: Ethical Implications." In American Association for the Advancement of Science, *The Genome, Ethics and the Law: Issues in Genetic Testing*. AAAS

Publication No. 92–115. Washington, DC: American Association for the Advancement of Science.

National Council of the Churches of Christ in the U.S.A. 1986. *Genetic Science for Human Benefit.* New York: NCC.

Rabinovitz, J. 1992. "Rape Conviction Overturned on DNA Tests," *New York Times* (December 2) B6.

Rabuzzi, K.A. 1987. "Family." In M. Eliade, ed., *The Encyclopedia of Religion.* Vol. 5. New York: Macmillan Publishing Co.

Russell, B. 1953. *The Impact of Science on Society.* New York: Simon and Schuster.

Schmeck, R.M., Jr. 1980. "Nobel Winner Says He Gave Sperm for Women to Bear Gifted Babies." *New York Times* (March 1) 6.

Seligman, J., Rosenberg, D., Wingert, P., Hannah, D., and Annin, P. 1992. "It's Not Like Mr. Mom." *Newsweek* (December 14) 70.

Trojan, J., Johnson, T.R., Rudin, S.D., Ilan, J., Tykocinski, M.L., and Ilan, J. 1993. "Treatment and Prevention of Rat Glioblastoma by Immunogenic C6 Cells Expressing Antisense Insulin-Like Growth Factor I RNA." *Science* 259:94–97.

Weber, M. 1958. "Politics as a Vocation." In H.H. Gerth and C.W. Mills, trans. and ed., *From Max Weber: Essays in Sociology.* New York: Oxford University Press.

Whitehead, A.N. 1925. *Science in the Modern World.* New York: Macmillan Publishing Co.

World Council of Churches. 1989. *Biotechnology: Its Challenge to the Churches and the World.* Geneva, Switzerland: WCC.

2

And Baby Makes Three — Or Four, or Five, or Six: Defining the Family After the Genetic Revolution

R. Alta Charo, J.D.

After four miscarriages, Adria Blum was ecstatic when her son was born four years ago. The child's father, Barry Chersky, comforted Blum in the delivery room during the many hours of labor.

So did Adria's lover, Marilyn. So did Barry's lover, Michael Baiad. Now the four Oakland residents, all in their 40s, share custody of Ari, a rambunctious 3-year-old conceived through artificial insemination. He feels sorry for other kids because they don't all have a Mommy, a Daddy, a Marilyn and a Michael. (Tuller 1993)

The "Ten O'Clock News" in New York City used to run a public service announcement in the 1970s that read: "It's ten o'clock. Do you know where your children are?" Perhaps it is time to update the message to read: "It's the 1990s. Do you know who all your parents are?" In the 1990s, we have a marvelous opportunity to rethink our prejudices concerning the definition of a family. Our emotional attachment to a definition based on blood, our modern tendency toward a definition based on contract, and our legal definitions based on fictional re-creations of the biological nuclear family are all ripe for reform and integration. The result could be an expansion in the number of adults recognized as having parental ties to a particular child, an end to unthinking opposition to homosexual or group marriage, and a flowering of classical liberal theory in which the role of government is to facilitate individual choice rather than shape it.

This chapter will review the inconsistencies in European and American legal definitions of the family. Following a description of the competing claims of gestational, genetic, and contractual relationships to preferential treatment in cases of contested parenthood, the chapter concludes that each type of relationship has been made to yield to significant nonbiological concerns. Thus, over time, biology and intention to parent have been sacrificed to the need for orderly transmission of property between generations, stability of marital units as the fundamental structure of social organization, and finally, protection of children's perceived best interests.

As it appears that social policy provides an acceptable reason to violate the integrity of parent—child relationships, this chapter argues that social policy could similarly be used to maintain that integrity. Specifically, the preference for heterosexual couples as parents is unwarranted and single persons, homosexual couples, and larger groups of adults may serve equally well as parents. Furthermore, expanding the definition of parenthood to permit all genetic, gestational, and contractual parents to be recognized simultaneously will spare the courts the task of identifying which adults to discard from the child's life. This abandonment of legal fictions—which maintain that a child has at most two parents of different gender, regardless of biological and psychological reality—is a recognition that law need not slavishly follow cramped visions of nature but can instead facilitate broader visions of justice.

The Genetic Model of the Family

The redefinition of "family" is timely for four reasons. First, the increased frequency of divorce and stepparenting has made traditional allocations of parental rights and responsibilities unworkable in light of the day-to-day experience of children living with "stepparents." Second, the frequency of single persons and homosexual couples seeking to parent has strained the two-person, two-gender model of parenthood. Third, the advent of so-called gestational surrogacy has clouded identification of "biological" maternity, thus for the first time opening the door to an examination of just what it is about biological parenthood that entitles it to such extraordinary respect.

Finally, the Human Genome Project promises to usher in an era of genetic exploration and invention (Kevles and Hood 1992; Davis 1991; Bishop and Waldholz 1990; Wingerson 1990; Committee 1988). As with nineteenth-century advances, this knowledge may well become the basis for profound shifts in public thinking and public policy, just as Darwinian evolutionary theory became the basis of Spencerian libertarian theory and subsequent eugenic social policy (Lewontin 1992; Nelkin and Tancredi 1991; Suzuki and Knudtson 1990; Kevles 1986). With increasing understanding of genetic influences on physical and psychological phenotypical expression comes the temptation to identify genetic coding as the ultimate expression of personal identity and genetic linkages as the fundamental expression of human relationships. But such a development would be overly reductionist and lead to unfortunate public policy.

The blood ties between parent and child have almost mythological significance in every culture (Chodorow 1978). They represent both the act of procreation and the physical reflection of the parent's body in the body of the child (Sorosky 1984; Bluestein 1982). The importance of genetic ties is confirmed by research suggesting that many psychological attributes may also be influenced by genetic heritage (Wilson 1978), although environmental influences may swamp these effects (Lewontin et al. 1984). "In sum," states one commentator, "it is only natural that our sublime and complex feelings regarding this issue reflect precisely the sentiment that law should preserve as a family unit that which nature has rendered genetically similar" (Hill 1992).

The emotional significance of that biological link became enshrined in religious traditions that grappled with death and the finiteness of humankind. Many cultures and religious traditions, such as Judaism, hold that there is no formal "afterlife." Rather, we live on through our children, a kind of limited, genetic immortality (Lifton 1983). Their memories of us continue our existence. And when the memories fail, a small part of ourselves, our genes and our traits, still persist. It is no coincidence, then, that Jewish tradition dictates that a man marry his brother's widow if the brother should die childless (Deuteronomy 25:3–10). To do less would surely be to condemn the brother to true death.

"The significance of the genetic connection between parent and child," writes one commentator, "undoubtedly is part of what makes infertility a painful experience. While adoption may satisfy one's desire to provide nurturance for a child, adoption cannot satisfy the yearning to create the child and to watch as a version of oneself unfolds and develops" (Hill 1992). And it is the very fact that many reproductive technologies involve relinquishing access to children who are one's genetic progeny that has led some to condemn the practice as "unnatural" or "immoral" (Krimmel 1983).

However, it is easy to place too much mystical importance on genetic connections. After all, there is no statistical genetic difference between the relationship of the donor and child and the relationship between full siblings. It is the added psychological aspects of parenting that give the parental/genetic connection such an entitlement to legal recognition. Nor should the fact that one's child shares one's genes become the basis for a property rights argument in which the child is, in some sense, "owned" by the parent. Not only is this a dangerous doctrine that long led to child abuse and child labor, it fails to distinguish between owning the raw materials and owning the creation arising from them (Hill 1992; Andrews 1986a; Scott 1981). The same issue has arisen with regard to the use of a patient's spleen cells in the development of a commercially valuable cell line (*Moore* v. *Regents*, 215 Cal. App. 3d 709 [1988]). Thus, the progenitors of a frozen, in vitro embryo may be treated as property owners (*York* v. *Jones*, 717 F. Supp. 421 [E.D. Va. 1989]; *Del Zio* v. *Columbia Presbyterian Medical Center* [unreported; New York 1987]) in some contexts and as prospective parents in others (*Davis* v. *Davis*, 842 S.W. 2d 588 [1992]), but at the moment of birth the offspring is no longer property of any sort (Glendon 1981).

Thus the emphasis on biological formation of families may overvalue the significance of genetic linkages. Further, it marginalizes some children and adults with a significant involvement in the family. It ignores, for example, the frequent presence in nonadoptive families of children with biological ties to only one of the parents. Such children, when unrelated to the marital partner of the mother, were deemed illegitimate, severely disadvantaging them and their mothers. The biological model of the family, with this overlay of insistence upon expressing biological relationships within a socially sanctioned, heterosexual marriage, resulted in the creation of a grand presumption, to wit, that all "real" families follow this model absent a formal legal intervention.

But some families had more than two parents. Some were parents by virtue of biology, a bond that cannot be broken no matter how many legal proceedings are used to push the biological parents out of the child's life. Others were parents by contract, who by virtue of marriage to the child's mother or contract with the state created a psychological, economic, and legal relationship with the child. But legal fictions were maintained, in large part due to the fear that nonexclusivity of parental status would lead to hampered decision-making among the adults and thus thwart state efforts to make parents the primary providers of services and discipline to minors.

Later developments in foster parenting and the explosion of stepparenting followed this trend. No third party could gain a permanent, legally recognized relationship with a child absent an extraordinary intervention by the courts or by the permanent withdrawal of the natural parents from the child's life. These biological, or "real," parents were given an almost unbeatable presumption in their favor when it came to contested custody and parenting cases, and when supplanted by nonbiological parents, they were made to disappear in order to re-create the illusion of a "biological" family. Thus this Western tradition dictated that there could be only one of each type of parent, although other societies freely experimented with polygyny (Strathern 1991).

The Contractual Model of the Family

At the same time, though, this seeming fascination with biology had a strong competitor—the need to find substitute parents when genetic linkages were missing or inconvenient. Adoption, a statutory creation not existing at common law (*Smith* v. *Organization of Foster Families*, 431 U.S. 816, 845-846 [1977]) though long taking place informally or with private legislation (Sloan 1988), is evidence of a strong social tradition that recognizes the purely social and psychological dimensions of parenting, even where these occur in the absence of biological ties. Yet, even with adoption, adoptive parents may acquire parental status with respect to a particular child only after termination of the parental rights of the child's biological parents, particularly those of the natural mother. The "presumption of biology" serves as an irrebuttable legal presumption that the birth mother of the child is its legal mother and that adoption can take place only consequent to a termination of the parental rights of the birth mother (Andrews 1986b; Aires 1962).

In early Rome and in other ancient cultures, adoption served a primarily religious function associated with ensuring that a legitimate male heir would carry out sacred obligations (Presser 1971). Even after the religious overtones vanished, civil law countries viewed adoption principally as a vehicle for perpetuating the adoptive parent's name and property rather than as a means of benefiting the adoptee (Presser 1971; Huard 1956; Kuhlman 1943). The English common law did not recognize adoption at all; England finally legalized it by statute in 1926 (The "Adoption of Children Act," 1926, 16 & 17 Geo. 5, ch. 29). In the United States, adoption began as a means for privatizing the cost of maintaining orphans. It only later became grounded in child welfare, and that welfare was generally defined as re-creation of a biological-style family unit for the child to enter.

A more cynical explanation, therefore, of the romanticization of genetic linkages between father and child, and the degree to which adoption is structured to re-create families with clear lines of succession from a single father, rests on the needs of men to conserve their property for the benefit of only a few children, those to whom they are truly related by blood and whom they have, in a sense, contracted to sire (Presser 1971).

Adoption as known today did not fully emerge until the mid-nineteenth century when general adoption legislation was introduced on a wave of social welfare reform (Presser 1971). Before then, child placement in this country was an informal affair. Upon the death of one or both parents, a child was simply "put out" for a suitable blood relative, usually designated in the decedent's will, to raise. Orphaned or abandoned children without family connection and too young for apprenticeship went to public institutions until they were useful enough to be either "bound out" (indentured or apprenticed) or sent to uninvestigated homes (Presser 1971; Calhoun 1917). Although some attention was paid to the child's well-being, placement mainly served to privatize the cost of the child's education and care, while providing inexpensive labor to the adults taking in the child (Laslett 1974).

By the nineteenth century, the economic atmosphere tempted many adoptive parents to take advantage of a child's labor without returning much by way of education and succor (Presser 1971; Folks 1902). Christian reformers, through religiously affiliated private agencies, began to shift the focus of their efforts toward the placement of infants and young children in homes where they would be treated more like family members than servants (Presser 1971). Adoption statutes soon followed suit, reflecting a slow shift in public attitudes from the notions of apprenticeship and service to the notion that child placement should primarily serve the welfare of the dependent child.

Modern adoption statutes are replete with statements that make it clear that their primary focus is the well-being of the adopted child. The requirement of many modern adoption statutes that prospective adoptive parents pass a rigorous screening process before the adoption is finalized illustrates this concern (OTA 1988). In the case of the out-of-wedlock infant given to strangers for adoption, society generally deems it in the adoptee's best interests to make the infant a full-fledged member of the adoptive family, as though the infant had been born into the adoptive family.

Furthermore, it is widely believed that an adoptee's retention of ties with the biological family can undermine the psychological aspect of this assimilation. Thus, courts have described the broad objective of adoption statutes as "giving the adopted child a 'fresh start' by treating him as the natural child of the adoptive parent" (*In re Estates of Donnelly*, 81 Wash. 2d 430 [1972]), in essence a "substitution of the adoptive in place of the natural family and severance of legal ties with the child's natural family" (*Crumpton* v. *Mitchell*, 303 N.C. 657 [1981]).

Thus, once created by statute, adoption was designed to use law to re-create the image of a biological family unit. It required that the biological parents be permanently removed from the child's life and the adoptive parents substituted for them (Minow 1991). It was not possible for the child to be adopted without the natural parents relinquishing all parental rights and responsibilities. Under law, they became legal strangers (Dempsey 1981).

Discarding Biological Relationships to Maintain Biological Appearances

The other important purpose to be served whenever deviating from biological definitions of the family was the preservation of the heterosexual marital unit. Thus, many states passed laws that created a presumption of paternity on the part of a mother's husband. Indeed, the husband did not have to be physically present at the time of conception (Field 1988): "If a husband, not physically incapable, was within the four seas of England during the period of gestation, the court would not listen to evidence casting doubt on his paternity" (*In re Findlay*, 253 N.Y. 1 [1930]).

Common law went so far as to deny the biological father the opportunity to assert his own paternity of a child born to a married woman (Hill 1992), although it could be asserted against him by the mother or her husband. This generally remains true today (Hill 1992), even though forensic uses of DNA testing now enable paternity determinations to be made with great accuracy (OTA 1991).

Thus, the biological progenitor of a child does not enjoy a constitutional right to establish paternity for his own pleasure or to seek any form of legal recognition of the relationship if the mother of the child is married to another man, even where he has actively sought to establish a relationship with the child (*Michael H. v. Gerald D.*, 491 U.S. 110 [1989]). The rule not only protects the integrity of the family but also legitimizes the child (Hill 1992). In this way, biological reality gives way to three strong public policy considerations: that a husband should not be cuckolded against his will; that an adulterer not have the opportunity to demand access to his genetic offspring; and that the appearance of a biological family unit be maintained whenever possible.

The conflicting interests here—the child's interest in having a recognized mother and father; men's interests in avoiding unwanted responsibility for nonbiological children; and men's interests in having access to biological children—are difficult to reconcile in a coherent fashion. Neither biology nor contractual relationships are the clear trump. What is clear, however, is that these interests must be sorted out within the paradigm of a two-parent, heterosexual marital parenting unit. The solution of declaring both the husband and the progenitor as fathers is simply not available. The Uniform Parentage Act makes these policy considerations quite evident.

Thus, the genetic relationship between father and child is considered secondary to the public policy of maintaining the integrity of "traditional" marriage and of rearing children, as often as possible, within such confines. Where no such "traditional" family is available, however, for example, when the child is born to a mother who is single or part of a lesbian couple, the law does permit the biological father to assert his paternal rights, even if he clearly stated his intention prior to conception to have no relationship to the child. This has been the case, for example, with sperm donors (*Jhordan C. v. Mary K.*, 179 Cal. App. 3d 386 [1986]). The Supreme Court has elevated this principle to a constitutional level (*Lehr* v. *Robertson*, 463 U.S. 248 [1983]; *Caban* v. *Mohammed*, 441 U.S. 130 [1979]; *Quilloin* v. *Walcott*, 434 U.S. 246 [1978]; *Stanley* v. *Illinois*, 405 U.S. 645 [1972]). Thus, a man achieves constitutional protection as parent of his child by virtue of the genetic relationship alone if there is no substitute parent and if he does not otherwise appear to waive the right (Bartlett 1984; Wright 1979).

With the advent of artificial insemination by donor (AID) services, courts and legislatures faced a fresh challenge. The procedure posed squarely the problem of determining whether genetic mixing without sexual intercourse constituted an affront to the marriage. Early on, courts held that it did, likening AID to adultery (*Doornbos* v. *Doornbos*, 23 U.S.L.W. 2308 [1954], *appeal dismissed*, 12 Ill. App. 2d 473 [1956]), although that trend was later reversed (Andrews 1984; Wadlington 1983). Second, courts were called on to determine whether genetic parentage, by itself, would be recognized under law as equivalent to legal parentage. As in nonadulterous situations of nonmarital sexual intercourse, the answer generally was "yes." Without a husband available to substitute for the genetic father, biological linkage created legal parenthood (Wikler 1992; OTA 1988).

But when the recipient of the donor semen is married, the presumption of spousal paternity comes into play, just as it does in situations of true adultery (OTA 1988). Over half the states have passed laws specifically stating that a donor is not to be considered the legal father of a child conceived by a married woman. But if the woman is not married, she is either denied access to the service entirely, or the donor is potentially considered the legal father, despite the fact that she is resorting to AID specifically because she does not want the genetic father to have a legal status vis-à-vis the child. The hope is illusory that the magical desexualization of conception by using a syringe rather than intercourse will yield the protection of the law against unwanted intrusions by the genetic father.

The Problem of Deceptive Appearances

At least with ordinary AID by married women, appearances of a typical, biologically related family can be maintained by discarding the inconvenient genetic parent. Not so with contract motherhood (more commonly known as surrogate motherhood). The wife of the genetic father, who intends to rear the child, is visibly unpregnant. Therefore, she is disfavored as compared to the biological mother (Andrews 1986b). For example, the New Jersey Supreme Court held that Mary Beth Whitehead (now Gould), the genetic and gestational mother of a child conceived with semen from Bill Stern, was still the legal mother of the child, the surrogacy contract notwithstanding. Bill Stern was the legal father, based on his biological relationship, despite the existence of Mary Beth's husband as a potential competitor for the title based on presumptions of husband paternity. And Mrs. Stern was left without any legal relationship to the child, despite the fact that she would be the child's custodial maternal figure (*In re Baby M*, 109 N.J. 396, 447–448, 537 A.2d 1227, 1253 [1988]).

This "presumption of biology" is premised on the ancient dictum *mater est quam gestatio demonstrat* (by gestation the mother is demonstrated). But ancient times had not anticipated the separation of genetic and gestational maternity into different, even commercialized components. For most of human history, the gestational mother had to be the genetic mother. If the two are represented by different women, however, which takes precedence?

The courts have confronted this conflict only twice, both times favoring the genetic over the gestational mother (Robertson 1989; Charo 1992). In the first case, *Smith* v. *Jones* (No. 85-532014 DZ [Mich. Cir. Ct. Mar. 14, 1986]), the proceeding was a "set-up" to allow the egg donor to adopt the child, and in accordance with the surrogate agreement, the surrogate did not contest the ruling. In the second, the court found that the definition of a "biological" relationship is that of genetic linkage (*Johnson* v. *Calvert*, No. X 633190 [Cal. App. Dept. Super. Ct. Oct. 22, 1990]).

The reasons for favoring a genetic model of the family have already been discussed. But there are arguments to be made that where a conflict arises between genetic and gestational relationships for women, gestation should prevail. These include arguments based on prenatal and postnatal bonding; the harmful effects to the birth mother of forcibly removing the child from her care; the physical involvement of the birth mother in bringing the child to term; and the uncertainties created when no hospital and no physician can securely hand a newborn up from the birth mother's loins to her arms.

It would be simple enough, then, to state that the woman giving birth is the sole biological, and therefore legal, mother. This maintains appearances. And it would effectively protect the egg donation programs that are beginning to flourish in states such as California, where women seek to use substituted gametes in the same way that men have done since the advent of AID. Those programs require that, as with sperm donation, the female gamete donor vanish into the mists of legal fictions.

But it would appear that this is not the approach of the California courts. In a recent gestational surrogacy case, a California appellate court held that a woman giving birth may be nothing more than a glorified wet nurse, and the child's real mother is the woman whose egg was used for the conception. A woman named Crispina Calvert had usable ova but no uterus. She had one of her eggs fertilized with her husband's semen and hired a second woman, Anna Johnson, to carry the pregnancy to term. When a dispute broke out after birth, an Orange County Superior Court judge ruled that the Calverts were the "genetic, biological and natural" father and mother and entitled to retain custody (Chiang 1993).

Johnson's attorney said his client wants only "a profound parental relationship" with the boy she gave birth to more than two years ago (Chiang 1993). Sensing that his best chance was to argue that his client was the "natural" mother, who is given preference under California law in cases of disputed custody, Johnson's attorney argued that "the term 'natural mother' means the woman who gave birth. Crispina is not the mother" (Chiang 1993).

A lawyer for the Calverts argued that state statutory guidelines for determining parentage in the context of paternity suits clearly mandate that the genetic parents be declared legal parents. "We can't deny that Anna Johnson had an important role, but does that confer a legal prescription that she is a parent?" asked the lawyer. "I think not" (Hager 1993). But Johnson's lawyer responded by arguing that "it is the relationship between the birth mother and her baby that is legally protected. It tortures the English language to say that a woman (like Mrs. Calvert) who was never pregnant and never gave birth meets the traditional definition of the term mother" (Hager 1993).

Nonetheless, the California appellate court upheld the trial court's conclusions, characterizing the woman who gave birth as merely a "foster parent" for the "natural" mother whose egg had been used. And the state supreme court, which has yet to rule, has reacted hostilely to assertions that the apparent mother, i.e., the woman giving birth, was indeed the "real" mother (*Anna J.* v. *Mark C.*, S023721, Feb. 2, 1993).

The continued viability of the "traditional" family unit, one that mimics what happens in nature, was very much on the minds of the California Supreme Court justices. Several seemed leery of the child ending up with a father and two legally recognized mothers. "Here we could have a genetic parent . . . and a gestational parent," said Justice Edward A. Panelli. "Is that the traditional family unit?" (Hager 1993). Chief Justice Malcolm M. Lucas wryly observed that it could prove awkward for a child to grow up with both a "mother" and a "genetic progenitor" (Hager 1993). And the court-appointed lawyer for the child argued: "The minor in this case can be served only by being raised in the traditional, two-parent family. To declare (Johnson) a parent would complicate the child's life—and has never been recognized under law."

This same fear of disrupting the definition of the "traditional" family unit led the New York State Bar Association's House of Delegates in February 1993 to reject a recommendation by the Special Committee on Biotechnology and the Law. The House defeated a resolution that called for expanding the definition of "parent" in the domestic relations law to include both the genetic and gestational mothers in surrogate births. Delegates, including several from the Trusts and Estates Section, were concerned that the proposal could have unexpected consequences in other fields of law. Several asked whether a child born through surrogacy would be entitled to inherit through both mothers. Limited New York precedent indicates that, unlike in California, the gestational mother would be the only woman recognized as the legal mother.

In the Johnson case, one justice seemed intent on examining the broader issues, asking whether it is possible to have two biological mothers. She also suggested during oral argument that one thing "seems to be forgotten in this tug-of-war . . . . What importance should be given to the child's best interests?" But the Calverts' attorney responded that the language of the Uniform Parentage Act, which defines a parent in terms of genetic linkages, already incorporates a child's best interests, i.e., that it is in a child's best interest to be considered the child of his or her genetic parents. The attorney did not comment, however, on the degree to which spousal paternity presumptions and adoption would therefore presumably not serve a child's best interests.

So What Is a "Natural" Parent After All?

The dilemma facing the California courts, who insist upon a single definition of "natural" mother but find that none will fit the needs of both egg donation programs and gestational surrogacy programs, is that they are trying to move toward a contractual model of the family without having fully abandoned the old biological models. In fact, it is the very power of genetic relationships that is driving infertile people and the courts to find ways to make surrogacy and AID more accepted (Wagner 1990).

One of the reasons given by Bill Stern for his decision to hire a contract mother was that his family had been wiped out in the Holocaust, and he wished to have blood relations with someone, somewhere. Egg donation is sought by women who want desperately to have the experience of being pregnant and giving birth to the child whom they will raise. AID is used so that women with infertile husbands can nonetheless have children to whom they are genetically related.

However, in order to make this possible within the strait-jacketed confines of the Western, heterosexual marriage, it is necessary that we simultaneously devalue the genetic and gestational relationships of the men and women who give or sell their gametes or their capability for gestation. Those biological connections must be considered less valuable than the contract these people signed when they became donors or surrogates. But the very fact that the infertile persons or couples who sought their services did not seek adoption to begin with testifies to the enormous significance of that biological tie. And the agreement the infertile partners of these biological parents have made to raise these children as their own testifies to the parallel significance of contractual agreements to take on these children as their own.

So if we insist upon a preference for "natural" parents, perhaps the definition of "natural" mother depends not upon biology but upon psychology—the intent to take the baby home. After all, what could be more "unnatural" than a woman who denies her own child? Consider two stories from Australia. In the first, Linda K. agreed to give a child to her sister. She gestated and gave birth to a child conceived with her infertile sister's egg. As she relinquished the child to the infertile sister, she denied feeling as if she was giving up her own baby girl: "I always considered myself her aunt." By contrast, Carol C. donated eggs to her infertile sister so the sister could become pregnant and give birth to children that the sister intended to rear. Reflecting on her relationship with the resulting children, who were her genetic offspring, Carol said: "I could never regard the twins as anything but my nephews." The births in these two stories occurred in Melbourne within weeks of each other (Charo 1992).

But if the definition of the natural mother depends primarily upon the intention to take care of the resulting child, then another California court decision, in the Moschetta case, makes no sense. Cynthia and Robert Moschetta hired a woman to act as a contract mother because Mrs. Moschetta was infertile. The contract mother, Elvira Jordan, was impregnated with Mr. Moschetta's semen and relinquished the child at birth to the hiring couple. Mrs. Moschetta cared for the baby at home for seven months, until the day Mr. Moschetta walked out on the marriage, taking the baby with him. In a three-way custody battle between Mr. Moschetta, Mrs. Moschetta, and the "surrogate," the California court promptly threw out the application of the one parent who had actually taken care of the child, day in and day out, for over half a year. Mrs. Moschetta, the court explained, was not the child's natural or (yet) adoptive parent and therefore had no rights at all. An argument can be made for the moral priority of this intended mother; but for her and her husband, and their desire to have a child, there would be no infant and no need for Solomonic decisions.

The Moschetta case is reminiscent of controversies concerning foster parents where the Supreme Court has said: "No one would seriously dispute that a deeply loving and interdependent relationship between an adult and a child in his or her care may exist even in the absence of blood relationship." Nevertheless, "the usual understanding of 'family' implies biological relationships, and most decisions treating the relation between parent and child have stressed this element" (*Smith v. Organization of Foster Parents*, 431 U.S. 816 [1977]). "In the end," states one commentator, "the Court appeared to create a distinction based on natural law, arguing that the relationship between foster parent and child is a creation of the state, whereas the biological relationship between parent and child is grounded in a 'liberty interest in family privacy [which] has its source, and its contours . . . not in state law, but in intrinsic human rights, as they have been understood in this Nation's history and tradition.'" While marriage traditionally has been the most important type of relationship, ascription of paternal rights also may depend upon the type of nonmarital relationship" (Hill 1992).

Shaping the Family to Conform to Public Policy Needs

Another possible explanation of all these seemingly inconsistent precedents is that courts are assigning parental status primarily to protect societal or child interests. Thus, the genetic father in the Michael H. case, who is both a psychological and biological father, is denied parental status because the mother's husband provides a substitute who fills important policy needs. Single women who become pregnant via intercourse or AID, regardless of the original intentions of the genetic father, are faced with court decisions declaring the donors to be the legal fathers. If these women are married, however, their husbands can substitute for the genetic father and provide the necessary camouflage. Egg donation poses no problem, as the egg donor simply vanishes in the face of the gestational mother who uses the egg to create a child for her to rear. And where competing claims are made to motherhood, based on psychological, gestational, and genetic factors, the maternal status is assigned to the woman who has two out of three characteristics. Thus, Mrs. Calvert is the "natural" mother because she is genetically linked and she was the first one who wanted the child. Carol C. may be genetically a mother, but she is not the "natural" (i.e., "legal") mother because it was her sister who wanted children and brought the twins to term.

Looked at this way, it is evident that there is nothing sacred about either genetic *or* gestational linkages or, for that matter, about psychological linkages. All are accommodated only to the extent that they are consistent with an overriding public policy in favor of placing children in homes with two parents, of different gender, and married to one another if at all possible.

This, then, opens the door to an explicit examination of which public policies are important enough to supplant our innate preference for favoring biological definitions of parenthood, and why we prefer when possible to place children in "traditional" homes, even at the expense of the interests of their genetic and gestational parents. While courts hold that primary custody should be granted to the parent who would best serve the interests of the child, these principles are not supposed to operate to remove a child from a fit parent merely to enhance the child's life chances (Ruddick 1979).

With regard to the great "gestation-versus-genetics" debate in the context of maternity, there are good policy reasons to favor a gestational definition. A majority of American courts, newspapers, and academic commentators have already adopted the term "natural" or "biological" mother to mean "genetic" mother. They write of conflicts between genetic and gestational mothers as that of "nature versus nurture," as if nine months of pregnancy is not biological, is not natural, but is some kind of extended baby-sitting job.

Perhaps it should not surprise us that so many confuse genetic links with biological links. After all, most of these judges and commentators are men whose only possible biological links are genetic. They will never have morning sickness in the afternoon or swollen ankles in the eighth month because there is a baby in their belly. They will never worry before drinking a second cup of coffee, lest it affect a developing fetus.

In a woman's world, pregnancy is indisputably a biological fusing of fetal and maternal bodies, health, and well-being. In a man's world, biology begins and ends with the DNA chains that link one generation to another. This rush to impose a male definition on a uniquely female biological experience could be considered a bad feminist joke.

It might be a joke if the consequences for women were not so frightening. Names are a form of classification that shape substantive rights. When Mary Beth Whitehead, a genetic and gestational parent, was called a "surrogate" instead of a "mother," the infamous Baby M case was already half-way decided, regardless of whether a pre-conception parenting contract should be enforceable. In the words of courts and commentators, a pregnant woman may be no more than a walking womb, a human incubator working on behalf of a future child. A month before the birth, one Michigan court declared that "plaintiff Mary Smith is the mother of the child to be born to defendant Jane Jones on or about July 1987." Imagine: a woman can be pregnant and already a legal stranger to the unborn child within her.

This country has seen prosecutors, hospital lawyers, and judges use court orders to stop pregnant women from smoking or to force them to undergo caesarean sections—all on behalf of a diffuse "societal interest" in the as-yet-unborn child. Think what could happen when it is not strangers but the "natural" and "legal" parents of an unborn child still in another's womb who are trying to ensure that the gestational mother, this "foster parent," does everything the way they would have done it. Will a pregnant woman's sense of fused biological well-being stand any chance against a legal property interest that others have in the fetus still within her body?

California's *Johnson* decision that a gestational mother is no more than a foster parent to her own child is almost without precedent in the world. Only Israel, bound by unique aspects of religious identity law, has adopted a genetic definition of motherhood. Every other country that has examined the problem—including the United

Kingdom, Germany, Switzerland, Bulgaria, and even South Africa with its race-conscious legal structure—has concluded that the woman who gives birth is the child's mother.

It is a conclusion that is essential if women are to maintain any degree of control over their own bodies during pregnancy. Anything less makes them ever more subject to the whims and coercive power of those deemed to have a superior interest in the child being carried. If, as the trial court judge in the *Anna J.* case asserted, it would be "crazy making" to recognize the reality of two natural mothers, then for the sake of women's rights and bodily integrity the one who is chosen ought to be the one who has given birth. And since the lesson to be learned from the cases concerning the presumption of paternity is that social policy can trump genetics, then all that is needed is a recognition that in this case a social policy favoring protection of women's physical autonomy is more important than either protecting the appearance of "traditional" family or the interests of the genetic mother.

Make Room for Daddy . . . and Papa, and Mommy, and Mama . . .

In fact, there is a better solution than choosing between competing biological mothers or between genetic and social fathers. We have already entered an era of "crazy making," where courts are re-examining the prejudice against polygamy when reviewing adoption requests by certain Mormon families and are granting visitation rights to stepparents and the homosexual partners of biological parents. Why not go further? Let us toss out legal fictions and recognize in court what has already happened in the physical world. Some children have three biological parents, not two. Some children have two biological mothers, not one. Acknowledging that two women are biologically related to the same child, that both women are "natural" mothers, does not necessarily determine who will have superior claims to raise the child. As every divorced parent in America knows, biology alone does not dictate custody.

Hundreds of children, most in San Francisco, New York, and other urban centers, grow up with multiple parents, usually due to arrangements among gay couples and friends of the opposite sex who were involved in the conception and birth. The lovers of the biological mother and father frequently take an active role in rearing children. Private contracts attempt to spell out relative degrees of involvement. Such coparents argue that their children, far from being confused by the unusual circumstances, actually benefit from being exposed to a wider range of adult influences. These families are more significant than their numbers suggest because they challenge the foundation of laws based on the heterosexual, nuclear family model (Tuller 1993).

A year ago, a group called Prospective Queer Parents was founded, which holds brunches that some participants have affectionately dubbed "sperm-and-egg mixers" (Tuller 1993). "On the second Sunday of every month, about two dozen gay men and lesbians interested in finding coparents gather to eat, chat . . . and scope out each other's genes" (Tuller 1993). "Our family arrangement is in many ways radical and visionary, since we're a bunch of four queers," one participant said. "But in other ways, we're a very traditional family—we value longevity, and struggling through for the long haul" (Tuller 1993).

Although the logistics can be complicated, coparents generally say that their biggest troubles come from a society and a legal system that fail to acknowledge the validity of their families. Consequently, the nonbiological mothers in coparenting arrangements often have deep concerns about their role and relationship to the child. One civil rights attorney working in this area says the law should be flexible enough to recognize that some families have three parents who all have legitimate rights, warning that it is the very rigidity of the legal system that can lead some coparenting disputes to end up in court, with lesbians and gay men fighting fiercely over custody and other issues (Tuller 1993). Thus, resolution of an upcoming Vermont case concerning the opportunity of a lesbian woman to adopt a child and thereby become a second, legally recognized mother is of great importance (Liley 1993). The probate judge ruled in June 1992 that Vermont's adoption law does not allow someone who is not married to a legal, custodial parent to become a second, adoptive parent of the legal parent's children. But Vermont's adoption law, last amended in 1947, contradicts itself and could never have envisioned today's families (Liley 1993). The attorney who represents the couple cites a section from state law that allows a single person to adopt a child. She says the mother's lesbian partner meets the prerequisites. However, a separate area of the statute reads that the parental rights of a biological parent are terminated once an adoption is granted. The only exception is for stepparents, a role that the biological mother fills but cannot claim because of the prohibition on homosexual marriage.

Perhaps it is time to take a great leap in family law. We could recognize that all biological relationships—genetic and gestational—are irrevocable. The emotional and medical significance of the bonds cannot be undone by signing a contract or adoption papers. The thousands of children who have wondered about the biological parents who gave them up for adoption or the sperm donors used to conceive them already know this.

At the same time, the voluntary social responsibilities we take on when we adopt children are equally permanent and no less profound. That is why so many adopted children, though they may wonder about their biological parents, take no action to find them. Forced by society to choose among various adults, these adopted children understand that the most important parent is the one who tries to stay around.

Why not give these children a break? Once a parent enters a child's life, whether by virtue of genes, gestation, or declaration, there is an unbreakable bond of psychology and history between the two. Crispina Calvert, Anna Johnson, Elvira Jordan, Cynthia Moschetta, Linda K., Carol C., and Mary Beth Whitehead are all mothers to their children, just as Robert Moschetta and Bill Stern are fathers to their children. Even for those whose parents are absent due to contract, abandonment, or involuntary events, there is a mutual tie of emotion, of wondering how the other is doing, and of moral responsibility. While courts and legislatures may see the need to determine who has a primary role in raising the child, there is no need to cut these other people out entirely. Indeed, from the child's point of view, it is simply wrong to do so.

In an age when courts have been forced to manage the untidy families created by divorce and remarriage, it is simply not enough to argue that it will be difficult to organize a regime of family law that accommodates the permanency of both contractual and biological (both genetic and gestational) ties. And having admitted already that stepparents and grandparents are indeed real family members, what legitimate obstacle remains to accepting the adults who enter family arrangements via group marriage or homosexual marriage? Surely we can be creative enough to create a new category, somewhere between custodial parent and legal stranger, that captures these relationships.

It has been said that you can never be too rich or too thin. Shall we add, perhaps, that you can never have too many parents to love you?

References and Additional Reading

Andrews, L. 1986a. "My Body, My Property." *Hastings Center Report* 16:28.

Andrews, L. 1986b. "Surrogate Motherhood: Should the Adoption Model Apply?" *Children's Legal Rights Journal* 7:13.

Andrews, L. 1984. "The Stork Market: The Law of the New Reproductive Technologies." *American Bar Association Journal* 70:50.

Aries, P. 1962. *Centuries of Childhood: A Social History of Family Life.* New York: Alfred A. Knopf.

Bartlett, K. 1984. "Rethinking Parenthood as an Exclusive Status: The Need for Legal Alternatives When the Premise of the Nuclear Family Has Failed." *Virginia Law Review* 70:879.

Bishop, J.E. and Waldholz, M. 1990. *Genome: The Story of the Most Astonishing Scientific Adventure of Our Time—The Attempts to Map All the Genes in the Human Body.* New York: Simon and Schuster.

Bluestein, J. 1982. *Parents and Children: The Ethics of the Family.* Oxford: Oxford University Press.

Calhoun, A. 1917. *A Social History of the American Family*. Cleveland: The Arthur H. Clark Co.

Charo, R.A. 1992. "Surrogacy in the United States." In S. McLean, ed., *Law Reform and Human Reproduction*. Hampshire: Dartmouth Publishing.

Chiang, H. 1993. "Surrogate Mother Custody Case Argued in State High Court." *San Francisco Chronicle* (February 3) 45.

Chodorow, N. 1978. *The Reproduction of Mothering: Psychoanalysis of Gender*. Berkeley: University of California Press.

Committee on Mapping and Sequencing the Human Genome. 1988. *Mapping and Sequencing the Human Genome*. Washington, DC: National Academy Press.

Davis, J. 1991. *Mapping the Code: The Human Genome Project and the Choices of Modern Science*. New York: Wiley.

Dempsey, J. 1981. *Family and Public Policy*. Baltimore: P.H. Brookes Publishing Co.

Field, M. 1988. *Surrogate Motherhood? Surrogate Fatherhood?* Cambridge: Harvard University Press.

Folks, H. 1992. *The Care of Destitute, Neglected, and Delinquent Children* 64–65. Salem, NH: Ayer Co. Publishers Inc.

Glendon, M. 1981. *The New Family and the New Property*. Toronto: Butterworths.

Hager, P. 1993. "Justices Cool to Orange County Surrogate Mother's Case." *Los Angeles Times* (February 3) A1, col. 5.

Hill, J.L. 1991. "What Does it Mean to be a 'Parent'? The Claims of Biology as the Basis for Parental Rights." *New York University Law Review* 66:353.

Huard, L. 1956. "The Law of Adoption: Ancient and Modern." *Vanderbilt Law Review* 9:743.

Kevles, D.J. 1986. *In the Name of Eugenics: Genetics and the Uses of Human Heredity*. Berkeley: University of California Press.

Kevles, D.J. and Hood, L., eds. 1992. *The Code of Codes: Scientific and Social Issues in the Human Genome Project*. Cambridge: Harvard University Press.

Krimmel, H. 1983. "The Case Against Surrogate Parenting." *Hastings Center Report* 13:35.

Kuhlman, F. 1943. "Intestate Succession By and From the Adopted Child." *Washington University Law Quarterly* 28:221.

Laslett, B. 1974. "The Family as a Public and Private Institution." In J. Skolnick and A. Skolnick, eds., *Intimacy, Family, and Society*. Boston: Little, Brown.

Lewontin, R.C. 1991. *Biology as Ideology: The Doctrine of DNA*. New York: Harper-Collins.

Lewontin, R.C., Rose, S., and Kamin, L. 1984. *Not in Our Genes*. New York: Pantheon Books Inc.

Lifton, R. 1983. *The Life of the Self*. New York: Basic Books.

Liley, B. 1993. "Lesbian Custody Case Goes to the Vermont Supreme Court." *Gannett News Service* (February 3).

Minow, M. "Redefining Families: Who's In and Who's Out." *Colorado Law Review* 62:269.

Nelkin, D. and Tancredi, L. 1991. *Dangerous Diagnostics: The Social Power of Biological Information.* New York: Basic Books.

Note. 1991. "Looking for a Family Resemblance: The Limits of the Functional Approach to the Legal Definition of Family." *Harvard Law Review* 104:1640.

Office of Technology Assessment of the Congress of the United States. 1988. *Infertility: Medical and Social Choices.* Washington, DC: Government Printing Office.

OTA (Office of Technology Assessment of the Congress of the United States). 1991. *Genetic Witness.* Washington, DC: Government Printing Office.

Page, E. 1984. "Parental Rights." *Journal of Applied Philosophy* 1:187.

Presser, S. 1971. "The Historical Background of the American Law of Adoption." *Journal of Family Law* 11:443.

Robertson, J. 1989. "Technology and Motherhood: Legal and Ethical Issues in Human Egg Donation." *Case Western Reserve Law Review* 39:1.

Ruddick, W. 1979. "Parents and Life Prospects." In O.O'Neill and W. Ruddick, eds., *Having Children: Philosophical and Legal Reflections on Parenthood.* Oxford: Oxford University Press.

Scott, R. 1981. *The Body as Property.* New York: Viking Press.

Sloan, I. 1988. *The Law of Adoption and Surrogate Parenting.* New York: Oceana Publications.

Sorosky, A., Baran, A., and Pannor, R. 1984. *The Adoption Triangle* 159. San Antonio: Corona Publishing Co.

Special Project. 1986. "Legal Rights and Issues Surrounding Conception, Pregnancy and Birth." *Vanderbilt Law Review* 39:597.

Spencer, G. 1993. "House of Delegates Puts Off Resolutions on AIDS Victims." *New York Law Journal* (February 1) 1.

Strathern, M. 1992. *Reproducing the Future.* Manchester: Manchester University Press.

Suzuki, D. and Knudtson, P. 1990. *Genethics: The Ethics of Engineering Life.* Cambridge: Harvard University Press.

Tuller, D. 1993. "Gays and Lesbians Try Co-Parenting: Families With 2 Moms, 2 Dads." *San Francisco Chronicle* (February 4) A1.

Wadlington, W. 1983. "Artificial Conception: The Challenge for Family Law." *Virginia Law Review* 69:564.

Wagner, W. 1990. "The Contractual Reallocation of Procreative Resources and Parental Rights: The Natural Endowment Critique." *Case Western Reserve Law Review* 41:1–202.

Wikler, D. 1992. "The Family as Social Construct: Dilemmas of Kinship Determinations in Artificial Insemination." United Nations University WIDER Institute Conference on Women, Equality, and Reproductive Technology. Helsinki (August).

Wilson, E. 1978. *On Human Nature.* Cambridge: Harvard University Press.

Wingerson, L. 1990. *Mapping Our Genes: The Genome Project and the Future of Medicine.* New York: Dutton.

Wright, J. 1979. "Caban v. Mohammed: Extending the Rights of Unwed Fathers." *Brooklyn Law Review* 46:95–121.

PART II

Privacy and Confidentiality Issues for Genetic Testing

INTRODUCTION

Collection and Disclosure of Genetic Information

Laurence R. Tancredi, M.D., J.D.

Protection of the privacy and confidentiality of patients undergoing genetic testing is becoming a major area of concern for ethicists, social scientists, and policymakers. Through the mapping of the human genome—expected to be completed sometime before the year 2015—a wide range of genetic material will be available for testing and diagnostic labeling. Already more than 1,400 genes have been mapped to specific chromosomes. Many single-gene disorders such as Huntington's disease and cystic fibrosis have been identified. Geneticists have identified the gene involved with colon cancer and are close to isolating the genes that are involved with other types of cancers as well. More complex conditions with multiple-gene involvement, such as mental illness, alcoholism, and heart disease, are being investigated with the goal of identifying markers that can be used for early detection of those predisposed to the illnesses.

Genetic information can be stored in computerized files and retrieved relatively easily with currently limited controls over their dissemination. Already efforts are being made to develop DNA databanks. The FBI is in the process of creating one such "bank" that will contain DNA fingerprints of offenders and criminals. Although this information will be used for criminal investigations, DNA specimens may be used for a variety of purposes. Furthermore, the concept of a DNA databank will probably be adopted in time by other social institutions for reasons other than use in the legal process. A health care institution may justify creating a DNA databank on the grounds that prediction of diseases offers some opportunity for early intervention and perhaps prevention of their more serious sequelae. An insurer may justify the creation of a DNA databank for enhancing actuarial estimates of population groups to develop benefit packages.

With increasing sophistication in our understanding of normal and defective genes, it may be possible in the near future to create a storage bank of biological information about an individual when he or she is born, which would provide an opportunity for early profiling of illnesses and disorders as well as behavioral characteristics. Genetic data that may be used to predict personal characteristics may also be used to predict the biological status of other family members, thereby extending the possibilities of invasion of privacy through gene analysis from individuals to their families.

Information about an individual's genetic makeup is highly personal and if revealed may impact significantly on his or her interpersonal and social life as well as benefits from social institutions—the workplace, schools, and the health care system. In many respects, such information deals with more personal issues than any other medical fact. A patient suffering from respiratory difficulties, for example, may keep others from knowing the basis for the difficulties, i.e., that it is viral, bacterial, or malignant in origin, but is unlikely to keep secret the fact that a respiratory problem exists. In contrast, the genetic makeup of an individual is for the most part hidden to others. Genes are essentially subcellular "invisible" substrates substantially responsible for an individual's physical and psychological characteristics. As such, they are generally revealed inferentially through external manifestations that may show up at different periods during an individual's life span. The exception would be where external signs of a genetic disease, such as may occur with a condition like neurofibromatosis, are revealed early to the observer.

The potential for prediction through genetics is currently believed to surpass prediction based on other biological data. This fact alone (though it remains controversial) gives urgency to the need for protection of privacy rights. In the case of an illness such as tuberculosis, it may become possible through the application of epidemiological techniques to predict the likelihood of a population group or even an individual contracting the disease. Once the disease has developed, the outcome may be predicted based on the severity of early symptoms and response to medications. Medicine has a long history of studying the course of epidemics and the prognosis of diseases. However, with genetics, "prediction" is at a higher level of precision. The factor determining prediction is inherent to the individual in contrast to general epidemics where the relevant factor is external, e.g., the presence of a germ, malnutrition, or congested housing. Prediction based on the presence of a gene or genes includes not only the anticipated morbidity and mortality from a manifested genetic condition (which in the case of Huntington's may be predictable at 100 percent accuracy if the afflicted individual lives long enough) but also the likelihood, not on statistical grounds alone, of a particular individual developing the condition in the first place. When a specific marker gene is present, prediction may occur years before the very early biological changes associated with a genetic disorder and does not depend on population patterns for contracting the condition.

Genetic information about an individual patient also affects privacy and confidentiality of other members of his or her family. The discovery that a patient has the potential for a genetically transmitted disease like retinoblastoma or cystic fibrosis means that other members of his or her family are vulnerable to being similarly afflicted. In the case of autosomal dominant conditions (an abnormality that can be transmitted when only one gene that constitutes an allele is affected), at least 50 percent of the other siblings from the same parents are at risk for the condition. This creates at least two major disclosure problems. First, the privacy of siblings who are susceptible to a genetic condition is arguably transgressed when one of the afflicted members of the family reveals that he or she is genetically vulnerable, simply because the inference is inevitable that the "gene" or condition may be in others. What limits if any should be placed on disclosure by a genetically afflicted individual?

Second, a sibling or relative who has been tested and learns that he or she carries a gene for Tay Sachs may not want this information revealed to others in the family. This situation clearly juxtaposes the individual's rights of privacy against the legitimate interests of others who would clearly benefit by having access to positive test results. Knowledge that a genetic condition is in the family would likely affect important personal and family choices. Some of the most important are whether to marry a particular person who may also be carrying the same defective gene; whether to have children and, if so, what precautions such as amniocentesis should be followed to prevent the birth of a genetically afflicted child; and whether a child already born should be tested for a disease that might not appear until later in life. The latter issue, especially where no medical intervention exists to alter the outcome, introduces its own set of issues regarding autonomy rights—the parent's versus the child's.

The responsibility of the physician or genetic counselor with regard to relatives who may be transmitting a gene introduces many critical ethical and legal issues. As the gatekeeper of genetic information, the clinician will be increasingly involved in conflicts of confidentiality and obligations to third parties. Patient autonomy regarding biological data is not necessarily an absolute right; compelling social reasons may trump that right, allowing for the disclosure of sensitive genetic test results. For example, might there not be justification to test an airline pilot where there is a family history of genetically induced sudden blindness from retinal detachment? There is precedence for balancing personal and familial autonomy rights in medical care where social need has been demonstrated. The history of public health in this country, going back to the nineteenth century, has involved discretionary and mandatory regulations requiring physicians to disclose information about their patients, such as the presence of a communicable disease or a gunshot wound and evidence of child neglect, to interested third parties. The Tarasoff case, decided in 1974, which involved the obligation of psychotherapists to warn and protect others where there is reason to believe they may be injured by a patient, has already been extended beyond psychiatry and further opens up the possibility of compromising patient autonomy regarding access to their biological—specifically genetic—status.

The scientific developments in genetics and the technology for storage systems of such information have considerably outpaced society's ability to respond with well-articulated policies that will protect privacy and at the same time address social needs. Although many social issues have been delineated since the beginning of the Human Genome Project, the complexity of interests affected and the diversity of social values involved necessitates that more groundwork be done on understanding their ethical and legal implications. Nonetheless, some policies are warranted even at this stage for strengthening legal protection of personal rights by establishing who may have access to genetic data and what circumstances justify overruling an individual's request for privacy and confidentiality.

The two chapters in this part address different approaches to the problem of privacy and genetic information. The first one, "Privacy and Genetic Information: A Sociopolitical Analysis" by Alan Westin, explores the history and development of privacy rights in the United States as these rights deal with the personal autonomy dimension of privacy as well as confidentiality (informational privacy). Westin explores the philosophical and legal basis for such rights as well as the functions that they serve for the individual and society. He proceeds next with an examination of the way privacy evolved legally and politically during a critical period of its development from the 1960s through the 1980s when landmark Supreme Court cases, like *Griswold* v. *Connecticut* and *Roe* v. *Wade*, gave constitutional body and extension to the scope of privacy rights. This section of the chapter involves his assessment of how the tradition of privacy will fare in the age of high technology, especially with the advances in genetics.

Westin continues with a review of surveys from 1979 that glean American public opinion about privacy. These surveys have emphasized the continuing distrust of Americans of centralized governmental institutions and the political process as well as the fear that computers and other technologies involved in the storage of personal data will be misused with the consequent loss of privacy. The chapter concludes with a summary of the important sociopolitical issues concerning privacy and an assessment of the struggles emerging with "new technologies and privacy claims," struggles that he feels involve power and ideological and economic relationships in society. In discussing genetic developments, suggestions are provided for what needs to be done to deal responsibly with privacy issues during the 1990s.

The second chapter, "Privacy and the Control of Genetic Information" by Madison Powers, provides a moral and philosophical approach to resolving many of the issues addressed by Westin concerning privacy and the potential benefits and harms of information disclosure. Powers begins his discussion by sketching a general framework for analyzing privacy from the perspective of moral concerns. This task is accomplished by examining the definition of privacy, the individual and social interests affected, the moral significance of these interests, the nature of genetic information as it relates to these interests, and, finally, the way these morally significant interests relate to privacy rights.

Having outlined an analytical framework for privacy and autonomy, the second half of the chapter is devoted to applying this framework to how genetic information should be handled by social policy. Three kinds of privacy rights are delineated that are important in shaping public policy. The first two rights come under the umbrella of informational self-determination. They are the right to control the information that is generated about a person and the right to determine the information that may be revealed to others. The third type of privacy right is concerned not with domination over genetic information but rather with defenses against government and its agencies when a person's control over information is not effective. In discussing these rights, disclosure is examined in the context of research and the need for privacy protection, especially with pedigree studies. The chapter concludes with a perception of the most important responsibilities of social and economic institutions to those potentially injured by disclosure of personal information.

3

Privacy and Genetic Information: A Sociopolitical Analysis

Alan F. Westin, Ph.D., J.D.

Since the end of World War II, major advances in physical, psychological, and information-processing technologies brought with their major social benefits some applications that challenged basic privacy conditions and traditions of democratic societies. While some observers rate the American response to these threats as too weak and see our privacy today as dangerously diminished (U.S. Privacy Council and Computer Professionals for Social Responsibility 1991), the United States has managed a largely successful adaptation and extension of our pre-1945 privacy values and institutions to the new environments of high-tech society, and we are now working in the right ways to strengthen those privacy rights in the mid-to-late 1990s. Whichever judgment one adopts, it is clear that public and elite concerns over preserving legitimate privacy rights in an increasingly scientific and technological age have become a well-defined and often-voiced sociopolitical theme in contemporary life.

It is in this setting that advances in biomedical research and anticipated applications through the Human Genome Project promise to expand greatly the levels of knowledge that society will be able to discover about individual genetic patterns. These new genetic findings are expected to be used for a wide range of medical and social purposes, with much value for both individuals and society. But, once again, our society also faces the need to anticipate the pressures that such a powerful increase in social and institutional knowledge about individuals, families, and social groups will pose for the privacy interests of people and the privacy balances of democratic society.

Fortunately, we do not start from ground zero in fashioning our anticipatory analysis and social plan for dealing with advances in genetic information. In fact, we have three major resources to draw on:

1. A helpful literature describing privacy as a social concept and identifying the social functions that privacy performs for individuals and groups in democratic societies;

2. A relevant model of social action, in the process by which American privacy concepts were redefined in the 1960s–1980s era to deal with the advent of new information technologies; and

3. A body of revealing survey data and trend analysis showing how the American public and important population subgroups view issues of informational privacy.

Describing each of these three resources and suggesting how they can be applied to applications of genetic testing are the foci of this chapter.

Basic Definitions and Operative Concepts Relating to Privacy

Most definitions of privacy agree on a core concept: privacy is the claim of an individual to determine what information about himself or herself should be known to others. This also involves when such information will be communicated or obtained and what uses will be made of it by others. In addition, many definitions of privacy would add a claim to privacy by social groups and associations and also a limited (largely temporary) right of privacy for government bodies (Westin 1967).

When we examine how the norms of privacy are set in any society, we need to have in mind three settings: political, sociocultural, and personal (material in this section is drawn from Westin 1989, 1967, 1965).

Privacy at the Political Level

At the political level, every society sets a distinctive balance between the private sphere and the public order on the basis of the political philosophy of the state. In authoritarian societies, where public life is celebrated as the highest good and the fulfillment of the individual's purpose on earth, the concept of legally or socially protected privacy for individuals, families, social groups, and private associations is rejected as hedonistic and immoral. It is also seen as politically dangerous to the regime. Thus, authoritarian governments keep extensive records on people and create procedures to watch and listen secretly to elite groups.

In contrast, constitutional democracies, with a strong commitment to individualism and freedom of association, regard the private sector as a major force for social progress and morality. The public order—government—is seen as a useful and necessary mechanism for providing services and protection. But constitutional governments are expressly barred by bills of rights and other guarantees of civil liberty from interfering with the citizen's private beliefs, associations, and acts, except in extraordinary situations and then only through tightly controlled procedures.

Privacy at the Sociocultural Level

This political balance is the framework for a second level of privacy—the sociocultural level. Environmental factors, such as crowded cities and class factors of wealth and race, shape the real opportunities people have to claim freedom from the observation of others. In this sense, privacy is frequently determined by the individual's power and social status. The rich can withdraw from society when they wish; the lower classes cannot. The affluent do not need to obtain subsidizing support from government by revealing sensitive information to authorities, while those in economic or social need must disclose or go without. (Ironically, though, the rich, the famous, and the politically powerful are also the people whose efforts at privacy are the most assaulted by the media, political rivals, government investigators, etc. And, in an age of virtually universal record-keeping and credentials review, even the wealthy and powerful become enmeshed in the all-pervasive data-collection processes of an information-driven society.)

At the sociocultural level, privacy is closely related to social legitimacy. When a society considers a given mode of personal behavior to be socially acceptable—whether it is hairstyle, dress, sexual preference, political or religious belief, having an abortion, or other lifestyle choices—it labels such conduct as a private, rather than a public, matter. This generally means that such matters should not be inquired into for the purpose of denying someone access to the desirable benefits, rights, and opportunities controlled by government or private organizations.

When society does not accept certain personal conduct but considers it socially dangerous, society is saying this is not a matter of "private choice" and does not allow the claim of privacy to be exerted for it in settings where benefits, rights, and opportunities are being distributed. Thus, debates over privacy are never-ending, for they are tied to changing norms of society as to what kinds of personal conduct are regarded as beneficial, neutral, or harmful to the public good. This makes some struggles over privacy unfold in moral, religious, and ideological confrontations with powerful interest group competition.

It is also true that demands to "regain" or "preserve" privacy are sometimes, in reality, campaigns for major sociopolitical or institutional change wrapped in the mantle of individual privacy rights. In short, privacy is an arena of democratic politics; it raises fundamental debates about the proper goals and roles of government; the degree of autonomy to afford sectors such as business, science, education, and the professions; and the role of privacy claims in struggles over related personal or group rights, such as equality, due process, and consumerism.

Individual Privacy: Four Basic States

Finally, within the political and sociocultural limits just described, claims of privacy are asserted by each individual in daily life, as he or she seeks an "intra-psychic balance" between needs for privacy and needs for disclosure and communication. This balance is generally a function of one's family life, education, and psychological makeup. It reflects each individual's particular needs and desires and shifts constantly in terms of life-cycle and situational events.

Four psychological conditions or states of individual privacy can be identified. Sometimes an individual wants to be completely alone, out of the sight and hearing of anyone else. This state of *solitude* is the most complete and relaxed condition of privacy. Solitude provides the opportunity for repossession of self and for thinking, healing, resting, regrouping, and preparing for reentry and reengagement in social life.

In a second situation, the individual does not want to be alone but seeks the *intimacy* of connections with confidants. The individual seeks valued and trusted relationships with family, friends, or associates with whom he or she needs to share sensitive ideas and emotions, receive help and feedback, and deepen bonds of mutual self-revelation and connection.

A third state of privacy involves defining some things that individuals do not want to share fully with persons with whom they are in contact and involves the creation of *reserve*. Either by personal explanation or by social convention, the individual indicates that he or she does not wish certain sensitive personal aspects to be discussed or noticed, at least at that particular moment. When that claim is respected by those around a person, the individual achieves the state of reserve.

Finally, in what is only an irony in nomenclature, an individual sometimes goes out in public to seek privacy. By going into public places and mingling with people who do not recognize him or her, the individual achieves the fourth state of privacy—*anonymity*. This is the condition of being seen or heard but not known. Such a condition of anonymous relaxation—in bars or movies, at sporting events, on trains and planes, or on streets and in parks—constitutes still another dimension of the individual's quest for privacy. Anonymous writings and other unidentified communications—a tradition dating back to the days of our country's Founding Fathers—also fall into this category.

Self-Management of Privacy States

In all these states of privacy, the individual's needs are constantly changing. At one moment, a person may want to be completely alone, in "down time." At another moment, the individual may want (or even desperately need) the companionship or sustaining presence of an intimate friend. Or the individual may want to "open up" problems or situations to a complete stranger—the one-time acquaintance who will listen to the individual's problems, perhaps offer a sympathetic ear, but who will not be encountered again and will not exercise judgmental authority over the individual.

Such changing personal needs and choices about self-revelation are what make privacy such a complex condition and such an important matter of personal choice. The importance of that right to choose, both to the individual's self-development and to the exercise of responsible citizenship, makes the claim to privacy a fundamental part of civil liberty in a democratic society. Without the power to decide when to remain private and when to "go public," we cannot exercise many other basic freedoms. If we are "switched on" without our knowledge or consent, we have, in very concrete terms, lost our fundamental constitutional rights to decide when and with whom we speak, publish, worship, and associate.

Competing Social Interests in Disclosure and Surveillance

So far we have stressed the importance of privacy to the individual in a democracy. However, every organized society, especially complex and technologically advanced ones, must provide for the disclosure of information necessary to the rational and responsible conduct of public affairs and to support fair dealing in business affairs. Democratic societies must also engage in surveillance of properly identified antisocial activity to control illegal or violent acts. Managing this tension among privacy, disclosure, and surveillance in a way that preserves civility and democracy and copes successfully with changing social values, technologies, and economic conditions, is the central challenge of contemporary privacy protection.

Authoritarian and Constitutional Traditions

From the earliest periods of Western society, disclosure—surveillance functions have been vested in five types of social authorities: (1) the employer—landlord, (2) the church, (3) associations to which the individual belongs, (4) local governmental officials, and (5) national regimes. In every historical era, as conflicts for primacy raged between church and state, town and guild, king and baron, or employer and employee, the individual's desire to be free from controlling surveillance or disclosure has been a part of these power struggles.

Looking back over two thousand years of Western political history, we can identify two broad patterns of privacy and disclosure—surveillance. In the authoritarian tradition—exemplified by Sparta, the Roman Empire, modern European nation-state monarchies, and contemporary totalitarian regimes—the exercise of extensive powers to compel disclosure and to conduct populationwide surveillance has been an essential part of the system. By contrast, in the constitutional tradition—typified by Periclean Athens, the Roman Republic, the English parliamentary system, the American republic, and modern democratic nations—basic limits have been placed on the powers of authorities to put individuals or groups under surveillance or to compel disclosure of information considered private or privileged.

The issue of privacy in historical evolution is complicated, since demands for privacy have often been a rallying cry for groups contesting for socioeconomic or political power in a given national setting. Even recognizing and adjusting for this reality, it is fair to say that no political system with a reputation for liberty in its time, or since, failed to provide important legal and social limits on surveillance by authorities. And, in the modern era, as each new scientific discovery and technology application has unfolded, adjusting the balance among privacy, disclosure, and surveillance has become a central challenge for constitutional regimes.

These definitions, individual dynamics, social processes, and political contexts will need to be applied as American society seeks to balance valuable applications of genetic information with individual and group privacy interests.

A Model of Social Response: How the United States Redefined Privacy in the 1970s and 1980s

The U.S. Privacy Tradition, 1787–1945

Despite uninformed commentaries that see privacy as a "modern" development in the United States, dating from the famous Brandeis article in the Harvard Law Review (Brandeis and Warren 1890) or from even later events, the United States actually had the most concrete and sophisticated legal and social concepts regarding privacy of any nation in the eighteenth and nineteenth centuries (Flaherty 1967; Westin 1965). Though the word "privacy" does not appear in the Constitution or the Bill of Rights, the Founding Fathers gave the American republic fundamental constitutional guarantees against unreasonable search and seizure, forbade compulsory testimony and self-incrimination, and secured privacy for association and religion in the First Amendment. Privacy rights in first-class mail and in census enumeration were written into early federal legislation. And, by rejecting internal government passports, elaborate government record-keeping, government spy networks, and other apparatuses of royal despotism, the American republic nurtured sociopolitical traditions that gave vitality to the constitutional and legal rules. Then, as new technologies of communication and surveillance arrived during the nineteenth century—such as the telegraph, telephone, dictaphone, and camera—the American privacy tradition was expanded to provide meaningful protection of privacy in those settings.

It was in the period from the 1920s to the 1950s that the United States fell dangerously behind in adapting its concepts to new social and technological developments. As urbanization, modern crime, and social experiments such as Prohibition arrived in the post-World War I era, a conservative Supreme Court majority refused to put police wiretapping and other new surveillance technologies under the same court-order constitutional requirements as applied to physical searches and seizures (*Olmstead* v. *United States*, 277 U.S. 438 [1928]). A sharp discontinuity developed in American law and social theory between the classic definitions of privacy and the new realities of personal surveillance and organizational record-keeping. While courts said that any new protections of privacy had to come from legislative action, no sizable constituency of Americans sufficiently affected by or concerned about updating privacy rights forced federal and state legislatures to modernize the American privacy rules.

The Privacy Crisis of the 1960s

This was the setting when an explosion of physical, psychological, and data surveillance technology applications in the 1960s transformed the privacy issue from a matter directly affecting only criminal and radical groups (and the small civil liberties community of this era) into an issue that suddenly affected over 120 million consumers, employees, and citizens. This transformation took four steps—early alarms, empirical studies, new privacy concepts, and legal—organizational action (Westin and Baker 1972).

By the mid 1960s, a series of books, articles, and mass media treatments dramatized the arrival—and unfolding uses—of micro-miniaturized listening devices, zoomar lenses, parabolic microphones, psychological tests, subliminal advertising, and the most sweeping in its implications, the capacities of new computer technology to collect, collate, analyze, and disseminate vast bodies of personal data. The early alarms documented the upsetting applications of these new tools and

then sounded a fundamental warning: With the existential limitations that had traditionally sheltered personal privacy deeply pen-
etrated by these new technologies, it would take a reformation of
privacy values and concepts, adoption of new legal rules, and strong
incentives for new organizational policies if the American privacy
tradition was to remain viable.

The early alarms in the United States and other democratic nations
led to a period of empirical studies and government commission inquiries in the late 1960s and early 1970s, with computers and privacy as the
most important element. These study groups developed a model of
technology assessment that worked well then (and is available to us still).
It set forth a pretechnology portrait describing how information was
collected, stored, and used by various sectors of personal record-keeping
in society before the new technologies arrived, paying close attention to
the social values served by that sector; the balances among privacy,
disclosure, and lawful surveillance already established there; and the
problems and societal conflicts that were present in the precomputer
era. Then, the studies closely documented how new information technologies were actually being used, for what purposes, and under what
conditions and rules, looking to separate the fanciful (and fearful)
predictions from actual applications and near-term trends.

Especially important in the empirical stage was attention to the
major changes in social and political values and interests that were
sweeping democratic nations in the 1960s and 1970s. New rules as to
equality by race, religion, sex, sexual preference, and cultural lifestyle
were being won by struggle in the United States (and some other
democracies); new rights of political expression and dissent were being
fostered by the antiwar and student-protest tides of that era; and new
consumer and patient rights movements were coming into full force.
Unless new rules were set as to what personal information should be
collected and used by organizational authorities to determine who got
access to the rights, benefits, and opportunities of what was now an
organizationally dominated, credential-based society, the sharply changing standards for such access would be controlled by the pre-1970s
information practices. Thus, the empirical studies took new social and
political values into central account when defining what threats there
were to consumer, employee, and citizen privacy rights in early and
potential applications of new information technologies.

New Privacy Expectations and Rules

From these studies we moved to new privacy concepts. In the
United States and most other advanced industrial democracies, these
took the form of fair information practices (the U.S. term) or data

protection principles (in Europe). In strict terms, privacy is one element in fair information or data protection codes—the part that says that only relevant and appropriate personal information should be collected by organizations with valid social purposes; that information should be handled confidentially within organizations on a need-to-know basis; that personal information should not be divulged outside the collecting organization without the consent of the individual or unless required by law; and that personally identified information collected for one known and approved purpose should not be used for other purposes without the knowledge and approval of the data subject. Other aspects of fair information or data protection codes deal with values other than privacy per se—accuracy of information, due process (individual access to one's record and opportunities to challenge or correct), and data security (an organization's ability to keep its promises of information confidentiality).

Politically, two things energized and made possible the privacy movement of the late 1960s and 1970s. First was the recognition by the majority of the public that access to jobs, insurance, credit, licenses, and other vital opportunities depended on making the new computer systems of public and private organizations responsive to new individual-privacy rights and meaningful due process. Second was the Watergate incident—a dramatic example of how misuses of information could threaten the highest (and the lowest) political and judicial processes of the nation. The Federal Privacy Act of 1974, indeed a generation of privacy laws, is Richard Nixon's legacy to the nation, not by his championship but by his electrifying example of how information power could be abused.

Between 1970 and 1990, two streams of legislation took up the fair information practices challenge. First, general fair information practices statutes covering all federal government agency record systems were enacted in the Federal Privacy Act of 1974, and in similar fair information practices, laws for state agencies were adopted in about a third of the states. Second, area-specific legislation was adopted at federal and state levels, spelling out privacy rules and applying fair information practices concepts to credit reporting, banking, education, insurance, cable television, video rentals, and electronic communications, with more limited statutes in areas of employment and medical records.

At the same time, the judiciary contributed important updating of privacy rights. The Warren Supreme Court enhanced privacy protection for writing, speech, and physical actions when it overturned the conservative *Olmstead* precedent of 1928 and ruled in 1967 that the Fourth Amendment protected the individual's "reasonable expectation of privacy," wherever the communication occurred and whatever the technology used by government agents to obtain it. And, with the right-to-abortion decision (*Roe* v. *Wade*, 410 U.S. 113 [1973]), the Supreme Court provided fundamental constitutional support for the personal autonomy dimension of privacy. (Unfortunately, since 1967 the courts have contributed a steady stream of poor decisions regarding informational privacy issues, a point that will be discussed later.)

The Current Privacy Environment

In the 1990s, the privacy scene in the United States is marked by a number of characteristics and developments that are important to our preparation for a privacy analysis relating to genetic information.

A series of Louis Harris/Westin national public opinion surveys (Harris 1992, 1991, 1990, 1979) document that privacy remains a significant social issue in the 1990s. Three-fourths of the American public are concerned about threats to their personal privacy; two out of three individuals believe that consumers have lost all control over the circulation of their personal information by companies; a majority of Americans do not think that existing law or organizational codes are adequately protecting their consumer information; and a majority of the public feel that the present uses of computers are a threat to privacy and that computer uses may have to be "sharply curtailed" if privacy is to be protected. (An analysis of the sources of these attitudes and their political significance appears in the next section.)

While significant attention was given to government invasions of privacy in the 1960s and 1970s, public concerns today focus largely on commercial uses of personal information, involving business activities such as credit reporting, employer use of drug and alcohol tests, direct marketing, new telephone services such as Caller-ID, etc. Some government issues remain, of course, such as proposals for national identity cards, multi-agency computer-file matching, and FBI proposals for preserving their wiretapping access to new telephone systems.

The U.S. Supreme Court until now has chosen not to take a leadership role in expanding reasonable expectations of privacy into the new areas of informational privacy and applications of new information technology, whether of data processing or of telecommunications. In cases involving banking records, pharmacy prescription records, and police circulars to businesses, the Supreme Court has declined to install constitutional privacy standards for government creation of or access to computer information systems, stating that these are questions for legislatures to balance, not courts. However, one case in the late 1980s involving a Freedom of Information Act demand for access by reporters to the government's computerized criminal history records produced a Supreme Court ruling that personal information that was open to the public in the locality, such as a police station or local court, took on

much greater sensitivity and greater privacy interest when it was collected and maintained in a central, computerized criminal history file
(*Reporters Committee on Freedom of the Press* v. *Department of Justice*, 489 U.S.
749 [1989]). Despite this pregnant ruling, however, and some important privacy rulings by state courts (including some under new and
explicit state constitutional clauses on privacy), the legislative and
regulatory arenas are more likely to be centers of innovation and action
in the 1990s than the courts.

In that regard, the mid 1990s will probably see the enactment of
another wave of federal and state privacy laws. These are likely to include
federal and state legislation updating the Fair Credit Reporting Act of
1970 and strong privacy guarantees as part of any national health care
program generated by federal law. We are also likely to develop organizational privacy guidelines for the national computer data networks such
as the NREN (the National Research and Education Network) and other
forms of interactive data and voice communication systems. Important
debates can be expected over the issue of an individual's property rights
in his or her consumer profile. As more comprehensive records of a
consumer's transactions, income, family life, and general lifestyle are
collected from business and public records by direct marketers and sold
for the key target marketing by providers of goods and services, more
attention will focus on whether the individual has any assertible legal
rights in that profile, whether in terms of requiring notice and affirmative
consent for such marketing uses, offering compensation to the individual, or at least giving individuals effective means for opting out of
those marketing uses.

Debates will probably deepen over whether the United States
should move from its 1970–1990 pattern of fair information statutes and
litigative enforcement to some form of federal advisory or regulatory
commission. Admirers of the European systems of data protection
commissions, with registration, investigative, and complaint-handling
powers, believe that the United States should have, at a minimum, a
federal body that would serve as a focal point for studies, hearings, public
reporting, and recommendations, even if the American public is not in
favor of a federal privacy body with regulatory powers. Critics of these
proposals cite opinion polls showing that there is not yet a public majority
in favor of such an agency, despite widespread concern to strengthen
privacy laws and organizational behavior. Whether the Clinton
administration's arrival will bring added support to the creation of a
federal privacy body remains to be seen. A significant influence on this
decision will be the final version of the European data protection
standards being worked on as part of "Europe 1992," the effort to
economically and politically integrate the European Community. If
those regulations make it extremely difficult for American firms to

process personal information in Europe or to move the information between Europe and the United States because the latter's laws and procedures do not meet the minimum data protection standards set by the European regulations, this could prompt business support for federal action that might not otherwise be forthcoming.

Sources and Dynamics of American Public Opinion About Privacy

Analysis of privacy surveys from 1979 to the present shows that the underlying causes of these public concerns are two continuing trends— (1) high distrust of government and other institutions of American society and our political processes and (2) generalized fears about misuse of computers and other technologies. These orientations are more powerful than any standard demographics such as income, education, occupation, age, political philosophy, sex, or race, in explaining and differentiating attitudes toward privacy as a general value or toward the majority of specific privacy issues (Harris 1990, Westin Introduction). At the same time, analysis of the survey data shows that the American public remains highly pragmatic rather than fixed or ideological about privacy rules and social benefits (Harris 1991, Westin Introduction).

■ About 25 percent of the public are "privacy fundamentalists," very worried about losses of their privacy and what they see as improper commercial and governmental demands for their data; they seek strong legal rules to forbid such data collection and use.

■ At the opposite pole, at 18 percent, are the "privacy unconcerned," people who give their personal information gladly to get commercial opportunities and benefits, support broad law enforcement access to personal data, and simply do not see privacy as a real issue.

■ Between these two camps are the 57 percent of Americans who consistently score on surveys as "privacy pragmatists." They care about privacy, but they also want access to consumer benefits; they believe businesses have a right to get information when they are asked to grant credit, insurance, or employment; and they see public-records disclosure and reasonable law enforcement surveillance as social interests also to be met. Basically, when the privacy pragmatists believe a valuable social purpose is being served *and* when relevant fair information practices have been applied and are being enforced, they will support such information uses and provide a solid public majority for such activity. When they do not believe that information is being sought for a valid social purpose or when fair information practices are not being followed, these pragmatists will see privacy as threatened and can be mobilized to oppose such actions.

In short, the battleground for the political and social defini-tions of privacy rights in the United States in the 1990s, and for any legal measures proposed, is essentially a battle for the minds and hearts of the privacy pragmatists.

General Implications of the Sociopolitical Analysis

As resources for thinking about privacy issues in genetic testing, the following major conclusions can be drawn about the historical, concep-tual, and sociopolitical analyses just presented:

■ Though it has been shown that privacy values and their protection are essential to individual dignity and societal progress in democratic and constitutional nations, struggles over applications of new tech-nology and privacy claims often involve basic economic and ideologi-cal relationships in society and become power contests.

■ This becomes all the more sensitive when democratic nations find themselves in periods of rapid social and value change, with institutions and social relationships in flux. Such changes, as in the 1960s and 1970s and again in the 1990s, put privacy balances into constant motion and require very adept and responsive studies and conceptual rethinking.

■ The keys to preserving a creative balance between privacy and social advances are the stages of social action used in the 1960s–1980s era— anticipative analysis and early social alarms; solid empirical studies; timely, but not premature, group and public mobilization; and well-tailored versus global policies and mechanisms.

■ In undertaking such social-action programs, some comfort can be taken in what thoughtful privacy advocates learned in the 1970s and have reconfirmed ever since—technology applications always take longer, are less unidirectional and focused, and are more mediated by organizational and social forces and interests than the promoters (and journalistic celebrators) of such new technologies predict.

■ Finally, while the power and sophistication of computer and commu-nications technology is clearly making many uses of personal data possible in the 1990s that were only wishful thinking in earlier decades, those powers also make possible many strong and creative protections of privacy. If we mean to do so, information systems can be designed that give each person more choices as to the uses or nonuses of data than were ever before feasible or cost effective and that control the flow and access to automated records more securely than was ever possible in manual or weakly automated systems. We can organize active, computer-literate guardians of privacy to monitor data systems and emerging applications with a timeliness and sophistication that was not available in previous eras.

A Preliminary Privacy Analysis of the Human Genome Project

What Are the Privacy Issues?

A successful Human Genome Project could supply purportedly predictive and socially usable information about individuals in the following four areas:

1. Individual propensities to contract diseases, with varying degrees of certainty and varying degrees of medical therapies available to moderate or overcome any such disease;

2. An individual's status as a carrier of harmful or defective genes, even though not personally affected;

3. An individual's propensity to engage in antisocial behavior, based on theories of inherited characteristics having effects independent of nurture or environment; and

4. An individual's likelihood of having various exceptional abilities, based on theories of superior inherited mental or artistic talents (see Reference List and Additional Readings, Section IV, for references).

Though there are disputes among genetic scientists about the possibility of genetic codes being found to produce some of these predictions, and much dispute about when such genetic information might become available in even the most likely future applications, let us take the future possibility of the first two outcomes listed above as the kinds of genetic information that should be used for our privacy analysis. The arrival of tests to produce genetic information in these two areas—individual propensity to contract diseases and carrier of harmful or defective genes (areas A and B above)—could challenge existing privacy balances in five areas, each harking back to the social states and functions of individual and group privacy summarized earlier.

1. *The management of intra-personal boundaries,* in which the individual decides what to know or not to know about himself or herself. Though there are some situations today in which individuals must submit to medical tests for certain conditions—to attend schools, qualify for health or life insurance, obtain some kinds of employment, meet a specific public health purpose (such as a venereal disease report or infectious condition emergency), serve in the military—the conditions for these tests are usually pinpointed ones relevant to a particular social

setting and the results not usually communicated beyond the sector involved. Any social program that would automatically test infants at birth, children at a selected point in schools, all persons entering the military, or anyone seeking public health benefits or payments would subject tens of millions of persons to a life-defining and potentially life-opportunity-limiting medical test.

2. *The setting of intimate relationships,* in which genetic information obtained from testing one family member reveals potentially sensitive or life-opportunity-limiting information about other family members—children, parents, siblings, or other relatives. While there are already some family or genealogical studies that can produce similar familywide data and some genetic tests of these kinds, such tests are not today in wide use, nor do they have the depth and scope that the Human Genome Project tests would produce. Who within a potentially affected family will be consulted and have the right to decide when a family member is tested, or, if an individual makes this decision, who will decide whether other family members will be told that such a test was done and its results?

3. *Confidential communications,* in which individuals reveal sensitive aspects of themselves to trusted and confidence-bound providers of medical and health services, health counselors, psychological and psychiatric specialists, etc. What will be the duties of such care providers—to prescribe tests or to share the results with other family members of the tested individual and with other health care providers—and how will the tested individual's choices be factored into the ethical and legal responsibilities of the professionals? How widely within the "health community" will genetic test results circulate? Already today, sensitive personal information (such as diagnoses and treatments) are provided by health care providers to the offices and computerized data systems of government and private health insurance and health program payers; self-insured employers; quality-of-care and professional-standards examiners; and organizations trying to control fraud, waste, and abuse in the health delivery system. Though these organizations have come to be termed part of the larger health care system, few individuals with sensitive medical conditions are comfortable today with the ever-wider circulation and database recording of such identified information.

4. *Qualifications for societal benefits,* in which obtaining or providing new genetic information could become a requirement for key benefits and opportunities of society—health insurance, life insurance, employment, credit, licenses, education, public assistance, etc. Which genetic conditions will become total disqualifiers for some of these life opportunities? Which conditions will sort people into two basic channels of life—the healthy individuals with access to the best jobs, insurance, credit, etc., and those "marked individuals" for whom second-class status will become a way of life? The right not to be tested or not to have genetic information

used for some or all of these societal opportunity or benefit purposes could become the next major privacy campaign, affecting tens of millions of persons and raising exactly the issues of social discrimination or opportunity that fueled the privacy campaigns of the 1970s.

5. *Social control and public policies,* in which standards for government programs and operations could be deeply affected by the availability of genetic information—in criminal justice functions (as already taking place with DNA fingerprinting); the operations of tort law; access to social welfare and public assistance programs; military service; government research projects; and many others. Will genetic test results about individuals be brought together into central databases, and used as a screening resource for a wide variety of entitlement, access, and investigative functions of local, state, and federal government? Since governments must operate under constitutional rules (federal and/or state), how will courts apply constitutional privacy standards to government's potential uses of genetic information? Will legislation be needed to set the detailed rules that courts often are reluctant to write?

What Needs to Be Done in the Mid 1990s?

If we take the social-action processes of the 1970–1990 period as our model, we can identify the steps that are needed to deal responsibly with privacy issues in genetic testing of the kind sketched above.

First, the early alarms phase has already started. Given the continuing sensitivity to privacy issues that emerged from the past two decades, and indeed, the institutionalization of sending early alarms, there has already been significant writings, congressional hearings, mass media treatments, and scientific self-searchings focused on the Human Genome Project. The ELSI program—Ethical, Legal, and Social Issues in genetic research and information uses—provides funds for the U.S. Department of Energy and the National Institutes of Health projects that have directly addressed privacy issues and will continue to do so.

Second, we are entering the key phase of empirical studies. The timetables and likely application roll outs of genetic findings need to be mapped out on a disease-by-disease and technique-by-technique basis, to learn what is coming, when, and how various facilitating or impeding factors are likely to shape these developments—costs, staffing, resistances, etc. Also included in this empirical phase is a review and application of social science findings about privacy functions and social needs to the specific contexts of genetic information uses. Finally, the empirical phase requires developing and conducting sophisticated public and group opinion studies, probably through the use of concrete scenarios to communicate to respondents the settings and uses of genetic information about which the survey will probe their views. As in the 1970s–1990s opinion studies, the search should be for the underlying factors and situational conditions that will influence public attitudes toward uses of genetic information, and whether, in this area, major differences will develop on the basis of demographics such as race, education, and income—in effect, class factors. These findings should be compared with public and group orientations toward other privacy issues, to test whether genetic information uses produce similar or different patterns.

Using these empirical studies, society will be ready to formulate basic privacy rules and guidelines for uses of genetic information as they become available. While the fair information practices principles are a good start, the special sensitivities of genetic information and its radiating effect upon family members will require the creation of some different norms and procedures. In this phase, it will be vital to sensitize and bring into active participation a wide range of potentially affected interest groups, from scientific and health professionals to racial, religious, nationality, and other groups whose members' statuses may be directly affected by some genetic information, to associations of groups already affected by the health conditions that will be the subjects of the early genetic information breakthroughs. It will also be vital to bring into these discussions a careful exploration of how earlier uses of genetic information by the eugenics movement led to many racist and antidemocratic programs, and the threat that "master race" notions could foster "ethnic-cleansing" approaches in our time.

Finally will come the time for framing and considering legal and organizational action. A few statutes and regulations are already in place that control how genetic information may be used for insurance and employment purposes, but these are clearly early and quite partial approaches. What should be the level of policy action— omnibus measures or sector-by-sector and even disease-by-disease measures? When should we prefer organizational codes and policies or industry standards, and when should we initiate legislation or seek judicial rules of constitutional or common law? This will be no easy task, since we may well need to reform major features of American economic, social, and governmental life more deeply than we needed to do in the 1970s and 1980s in framing and installing the first and second generations of fair information practices laws and codes. For example, the arrival of genetic information of the depth many consider likely could require basic issues such as these to be reconsidered: How will we redefine the ethical and legal responsibilities of various health care providers and counselors for testing and the resulting use or suppression of genetic information? What new definitions will be adopted as to informed and voluntary consent and individual access to and control over genetic-information databanks?

Some Parting Reflections

An awareness of the history and role of privacy in Western political development suggests that applications of genetic information will not suddenly transform our handling of health, disease, and human development in American society in the next two decades. There are likely to be gradual applications of genetic testing, shaped and filtered through the existing institutional, economic, and social structures and values of society. And, we are likely to emerge from the social-action processes of the 1990s on privacy issues and genetic testing, as we did from the 1970–1990 era, with an updated and sociopolitically reflective framework for balancing privacy interests and medical/health progress in what many see as a new age of genetic knowledge.

References and Additional Reading

I. General Social Science and Analytic Works on Privacy

Barnes, J.A. 1979. *Who Should Know What? Social Science, Privacy and Ethics.* New York: Cambridge University Press.

Bok, S. 1982. *Secrets: On the Ethics of Concealment and Revelation.* New York: Pantheon Books Inc.

Brill, A. 1990. *Nobody's Business: Paradoxes of Privacy.* Reading, MA: Addison-Wesley.

Flaherty, D.H. 1989. *Protecting Privacy in Surveillance Societies: The Federal Republic of Germany, Sweden, France, Canada, and the United States.* Chapel Hill: University of North Carolina Press.

Flaherty, D.H. 1967. *Privacy in Colonial New England.* Charlottesville: University Press of Virginia.

Fried, C. 1968. "Privacy." *Yale Law Journal* 77:475.

Hixson, R.F. 1987. *Privacy in a Public Society: Human Rights in Conflict.* New York: Oxford University Press.

Inness, J.C. 1992. *Privacy, Intimacy, and Isolation.* New York: Oxford University Press.

Lewin, T. 1991. "In Search of the Source of the Right to Privacy." *New York Times* (September 14) A, 7:5.

Linowes, D.F. 1989. *Privacy in America: Is Your Private Life in the Public Eye?* Urbana: University of Illinois Press.

Miller, A.R. 1968. "Personal Privacy in the Computer Age." *Michigan Law Review* 67:1089.

Moore, B. 1984. *Privacy: Studies in Social and Cultural History.* New York: Pantheon Books Inc.

O'Brien, D.M. 1979. *Privacy, Law, and Public Policy.* New York: Praeger.

Pennock, J.R. and Chapman, J.W., eds. 1971. *Nomos XIII: Privacy.* New York: Atherton Press.

Posner, R. 1978a. "An Economic Theory of Privacy." *Regulation* 2:19.

Posner, R. 1978b. "The Right of Privacy." *Georgia Law Review* 12:393.

Privacy Protection Study Commission (U.S. Government). 1977. *Personal Privacy in an Information Society: The Report of the Privacy Protection Study Commission.* Washington, DC: U.S. Government Printing Office.

Prosser, W.L. 1960. "Privacy." *California Law Review* 48:383.

Simitis, S. 1987. "Reviewing Privacy in an Information Society." *University of Pennsylvania Law Review* 135:707.

Wacks, R. 1989. *Personal Information: Privacy and the Law.* New York: Oxford University Press.

Warren, S.D and Brandeis, L.D. 1890. "The Right to Privacy." *Harvard Law Review* 4:193.

Westin, A.F. 1967. *Privacy and Freedom.* New York: Atheneum.

Westin, A.F. 1965. "Privacy in Western History: From the Age of Pericles to the American Republic." Ph.D. diss., Harvard University.

Young, J.B., ed. 1978. *Privacy.* New York: Wiley.

II. Privacy and Databanks

Celis, W., III. 1992. "As Computers Begin to Track Drugs, Fears of Abuse Arise." *New York Times* (January 17) A, 12:3.

de Gorgey, A. 1990. "The Advent of DNA Databanks: Implications for Information Privacy." *American Journal of Law & Medicine* 16:381–398.

Flaherty, D.H. 1979. *Privacy and Government Data Banks: An International Perspective.* London: Mansell.

Graham, J.P. 1987. "Privacy, Computers, and the Commercial Dissemination of Personal Information." *Texas Law Review* 65:1395.

International Chamber of Commerce. 1981. *A Business Guide to Privacy and Data Protection Legislation.* Paris: ICC Publishing.

Lee, S.Y.W. 1983. *Databanks: A Selected Bibliography of Articles and Books.* Monticello, IL: Vance Bibliographies.

Longobardi, J.M. 1989. "DNA Fingerprinting and the Need For a National Data Base." *Fordham Urban Law Journal* 17:323.

Marchand, D.A. 1980. *The Politics of Privacy, Computers, and Criminal Justice Records: Controlling the Social Costs of Technological Change.* Arlington, VA: Information Resources Press.

Miller, A.R. 1971. *The Assault on Privacy: Computers, Data Banks, and Dossiers.* Ann Arbor: University of Michigan.

Miller, M.W. 1992. "Data Tap: Patients' Records Are Treasure Trove for Budding Industry." *Wall Street Journal* (February 27) A, 1:6.

Moffat, S. 1992. "Plan for DNA Database Assailed." *Los Angeles Times* (January 16) A5:3.

Rubin, M.R. 1988. *Private Rights, Public Wrongs: The Computer and Personal Privacy.* Norwood, NJ: Ablex.

Rule, J., McAdams, D., Stearns, L., and Uglow, D. 1980. *The Politics of Privacy: Planning for Personal Data Systems as Powerful Technologies.* New York: Elsevier.

Shapiro, E.D. and Weinberg, M.L. 1990. "DNA Databanking: The Dangerous Erosion of Privacy." *Cleveland State Law Review* 38:455.

Shattuck, J. 1984. "In the Shadow of 1984: National Identification Systems, Computer-Matching, and Privacy in the United States." *Hastings Law Journal* 35:991.

U.S. Privacy Council and Computer Professionals for Social Responsibility. 1991. "Privacy Law in the United States: Failing To Make the Grade."

Westin, A.F. 1976. *Computers, Health Records, and Citizen Rights.* New York: Petrocelli.

Westin, A.F. and Baker, M.A. 1972. *Databanks in a Free Society.* New York: Quadrangle Books.

III. Privacy Surveys

Gandy, O. 1989. "The Preference for Privacy: In Search of the Social Locations of Privacy Orientations."

Harris, L. 1983. *The Road After 1984: The Impact of Technology on Society.* New York: Louis Harris and Associates.

Harris, L. and Westin, A.F. 1992. *Harris-Equifax Consumer Privacy Survey 1992.* New York: Louis Harris and Associates.

Harris, L. and Westin, A.F. 1991. *Harris-Equifax Consumer Privacy Survey 1991.* New York: Louis Harris and Associates.

Harris, L. and Westin, A.F. 1990. *The Equifax Report on Consumers in the Information Age.* New York: Louis Harris and Associates.

Harris, L. and Westin, A.F. 1979. *The Dimensions of Privacy.* New York: Louis Harris and Associates.

Katz, J.E. and Tassone, A.R. 1990. "The Polls—A Report: Public Opinion Trends: Privacy & Information Technology." *Public Opinion Quarterly* 54:125.

McClosky, H. and Brill, A. 1983. *Dimensions of Tolerance: What Americans Believe About Civil Liberties.* New York: Russell Sage Foundation.

IV. Genetics and Related Biomedical Applications

Ad Hoc Committee on DNA Technology (American Society of Human Genetics). 1987. *DNA Banking and DNA Analysis: Points to Consider* (October 9).

Aiken, H.D.and Hilton, B., eds. (John E. Fogarty International Center for Advanced Study in the Health Sciences). 1973. *Ethical Issues in Human Genetics: Genetic Counseling and the Use of Genetic Knowledge.* New York: Plenum Press.

American Association for the Advancement of Science. 1992. *The Genome, Ethics, and the Law: Issues in Genetic Testing.* AAAS Publication No. 92–115. Washington, DC: American Association for the Advancement of Science.

American Council of Life Insurance (Health Insurance Association of America). 1991. *Report of the ACLI-HIAA Task Force on Genetic Testing: 1991.*

American Council of Life Insurance Subcommittee on Privacy Legislation (American Council of Life Insurance). 1990. *Genetic Information and Insurance: Confidentiality Concerns and Recommendations* (October 30).

Ballantyne, J., Sensabaugh, G., and Witkowski, J., eds. 1989. *DNA Technology and Forensic Science.* Banbury Report 32. Plainview, NY: Cold Spring Harbor Laboratory Press.

Brostoff, S. 1992. "CEOs: Defend Genetic Test Use in Underwriting." *National Underwriter* (April 4).

Brown, D. 1991. "Individual 'Genetic Privacy' Seen as Threatened." *Washington Post* (October 20) A6, col.1.

Brown, R.S. and Marshall, K., eds. (The Council of State Governments). 1992. *Advances in Genetic Information: A Guide for State Policy Makers.* Lexington, KY: The Council of State Governments.

Brownlee, S. 1992. "Courtroom Genetics." *U.S. News & World Report* (January 27) 112:50.

Cowan, R.S. 1992. "Genetic Technology and Reproductive Choice: An Ethics for Autonomy." In D.J. Kevles and L. Hood, eds., *The Code of Codes: Scientific and Social Issues in the Human Genome Project.* Cambridge: Harvard University Press.

Draper, E. 1991. *Risky Business: Genetic Testing and Exclusionary Practices in the Hazardous Workplace.* Cambridge: Cambridge University Press.

Garfinkel, S.L. 1991a. "Identifying Criminal Suspects by Genetic Samples." *Privacy Journal* 17(6):4.

Garfinkel, S.L. 1991b. "Insurers Take an Interest in Genetic Findings." *Privacy Journal* 17(6):5.

Greely, H.T. 1992. "Health Insurance, Employment Discrimination, and the Genetics Revolution." In D.J. Kevles and L. Hood, eds., *The Code of Codes: Scientific and Social Issues in the Human Genome Project.* Cambridge: Harvard University Press.

Gruson, L. 1992. "Gains in Deciphering Genes Set Off Effort to Guard Data Against Abuses." *New York Times* (April 22) C, 12:4.

House Committee on Government Operations (U.S. Congress). 1992. *Designing Genetic Information Policy: The Need for an Independent Policy Review of the Ethical, Legal, and Social Implications of the Human Genome Project (16th report).* Washington, DC: U.S. Government Printing Office (Rept. #102–478).

Joyce, C. 1990. "Your Genome in Their Hands (the Human Genome Project and ethics)." *New Scientist* 127:52.

Kevles, D.J. and Hood, L., eds. 1992. *The Code of Codes: Scientific and Social Issues in the Human Genome Project.* Cambridge: Harvard University Press.

Knoppers, B.M. and Laberge, C.M., eds. (Quebec Network of Genetic Medicine and the New England Regional Screening Program). 1990. *Genetic Screening: From Newborns to DNA Typing.* Proceedings of the "Workshop on Genetic Screening." October 13–14, 1989. La Sapiniere, Quebec (Canada). New York: Elsevier Science.

Leary, W.E. 1992. "Genetic Record to be Kept on Members of Military." *New York Times* (January 12) 1, 15:1.

Miller, S.K. 1990. "Genetic Privacy Makes Strange Bedfellows (W. French Anderson and Jeremy Rifkin Support Congressional Bill)." *Science* 249:1368.

Milunsky, A. and Annas, G.J., eds. (American Society of Law and Medicine and the Boston University Schools of Medicine, Law, and Public Health). 1985. *Genetics and Law III.* Proceedings of the "National Symposium on Genetics and the Law." April 2–4, 1984; Boston, MA. New York: Plenum Press.

Nelkin, D. 1992. "The Social Power of Genetic Information." In D.J. Kevles and L. Hood, eds., *The Code of Codes: Scientific and Social Issues in the Human Genome Project.* Cambridge: Harvard University Press.

Nelkin, D. and Tancredi, L. 1989. *Dangerous Diagnostics: The Social Power of Biological Information.* New York: Basic Books.

Office of Technology Assessment (U.S. Congress). 1990. *Genetic Monitoring and Screening in the Workplace: Contractor Documents.* Washington, DC: U.S. Government Printing Office.

Office of Technology Assessment (U.S. Congress). 1990. *Genetic Witness: Forensic Uses of DNA Tests.* Washington, DC: U.S. Government Printing Office.

Privacy Commissioner of Canada. 1992. *Genetic Testing and Privacy.* Ottawa, Ontario (Canada): Minister of Supply and Services.

Rothstein, M.A., ed. 1991. *Legal and Ethical Issues Raised by the Human Genome Project.* Health Law and Policy Institute. Proceedings of the Conference Held in Houston, Texas, March 7–9, 1991. Houston: University of Houston.

Shapiro, R. 1991. *The Human Blueprint: The Race to Unlock the Secrets of Our Genetic Script.* New York: St. Martin's Press.

Subcommittee on Government Information, Justice, & Agriculture; House Committee on Government Operations (U.S. Congress). 1992. *Domestic and International Data Protection Issues.* Washington, DC: U.S. Government Printing Office.

Sugawara, S. 1992. "Biotech Debate: Who Will Read the Gene Maps?" *Washington Post* (July 5) H1, col. 1.

Wertz, D.C. and Fletcher, J.C. 1989. "Disclosing Genetic Information: Who Should Know?" *Technology Review* 92:22–23.

Westin, A.F. 1989. "A Privacy Analysis of the Use of DNA Techniques as Evidence in Courtroom Proceedings." In J. Ballantyne, G. Sensabaugh, and J. Witkowski, eds., *DNA Technology and Forensic Science*. Banbury Report 32. Plainview, NY: Cold Spring Harbor Laboratory Press.

Woo, J. and Naik, G. 1992. "Legal Beat: Police Like Genetic Data Banks, but Critics Question Validity." *Wall Street Journal* (July 28) B 1:5.

V. Surveys on Genetics

Fletcher, J.C. and Wertz, D.C. 1990. "Ethics, Law, and Medical Genetics: After the Human Genome Is Mapped." *Emory Law Journal* 39:747.

Harris, Louis and Associates. 1992. *Americans' Knowledge of and Attitudes Toward Genetic Testing and Gene Therapy*. New York: Louis Harris and Associates.

Harris, Louis and Associates. 1986. *Public Attitudes Toward Science, Biotechnology, and Genetic Engineering*. New York: Louis Harris and Associates.

Macer, D.R.J. 1992. *Attitudes to Genetic Engineering: Japanese and International Comparisons*. Christchurch, NZ: Eubois Ethics Institute.

Singer, E. 1992. "Public Attitudes Toward Genetic Screening in the Workplace."

Singer, E. 1991. "Public Attitudes Toward Genetic Testing." *Population Research and Policy Review 10*. Netherlands: Kluwer Academic.

VI. Selected Legal Perspectives on Privacy and Genetics

Adelman, C.S. 1981. "The Constitutionality of Mandatory Genetic Screening Statutes." *Case Western Reserve Law Review* 31:897.

Andrews, L.B. 1991. "Legal Aspects of Genetic Information." *Yale Journal of Biology and Medicine* 64(1):29.

Andrews, L.B. and Jaeger, A.S. 1991. "Confidentiality of Genetic Information in the Workplace." *American Journal of Law and Medicine* 17:75.

Annas, G.J. and Elias, S., eds. 1992. *Gene Mapping: Using Law and Ethics as Guides*. New York: Oxford University Press.

Damme, C.J. 1982. "Controlling Genetic Disease Through Law." *U.C. Davis Law Review* 15:801.

Diamond, A.L. 1983. "Genetic Testing in Employment Situations: A Question of Worker Rights." *Journal of Legal Medicine* 4:231.

Doot, G.M. 1991. "The Secrets of the Genome Revealed: Threats to Genetic Privacy." *Wayne Law Review* 37:1615.

Eisenberg, R.S. 1990. "Patenting the Human Genome." *Emory Law Journal* 39:721.

Gellman, R.M. 1984. "Prescribing Privacy: The Uncertain Role of the Physician in the Protection of Privacy." *North Carolina Law Review* 62:255.

Gevers, J.K. 1988. "Genetic Testing: The Legal Position of Relatives of Test Subjects." *Medicine & Law* 7:161.

Gostin, L. 1991. "Genetic Discrimination: The Use of Genetically Based Diagnostic and Prognostic Tests by Employers and Insurers." *American Journal of Law & Medicine* 17:109.

Knoppers, B.M. 1986. "Genetic Information and the Law: Constraints, Liability and Rights." *Canadian Medical Association Journal* 135:1257.

Knoppers, B.M. and Laberge, C.M. 1989. "DNA Sampling and Informed Consent." *Canadian Medical Association Journal* 140:1023.

Lander, E. 1992. "DNA Fingerprinting: Science, Law, and the Ultimate Identifier." In D.J. Kevles and L. Hood, eds., *The Code of Codes: Scientific and Social Issues in the Human Genome Project.* Cambridge: Harvard University Press.

Reilly, P.R. 1991. "Rights, Privacy, and Genetic Screening." *Yale Journal of Biology & Medicine* 64:43.

Riskin, L.L. and Reilly, P.R. 1977. "Remedies for Improper Disclosure of Genetic Data." *Rutgers-Camden Law Journal* 8:480.

Sherman, R. 1992. "DNA Is On Trial Yet Again." *National Law Journal* (March 16) 1.

Sherman, R. 1991. "Employer Use of Genetic Tests to be Restricted." *National Law Journal* (November 25) 15.

4

Privacy and the Control of Genetic Information

Madison Powers, J.D., D. Phil.

The prospects of extensive collection, storage, and transmission of genetic information raise new and troubling issues of privacy. Many of these concerns can be traced to the vast array of potential uses for genetic information and to the fear that the proliferation of such information will result in social stigma, loss of economic and social opportunities, and loss of highly valued freedoms. Because the potential uses of genetic information are numerous and diverse, the inventory of potential benefits and harms will vary depending on context, and the best strategies for the protection and promotion of privacy will be a function of those contextual differences. The aim of this chapter is to present one philosophical approach to the resolution of such issues.

The first section outlines a general framework for the moral analysis of privacy issues. Any discussion of privacy must start from the fact that privacy theories and their applications are matters of considerable academic and public controversy. For example, critics have raised doubts about privacy, either as a legal doctrine or, more fundamentally, as a coherent philosophical category for understanding the moral issues at stake in practical controversies (Parent 1983). Other critics have argued that social policies and legal doctrines designed to ensure individual privacy can impede medical and scientific research, prevent the implementation of comprehensive strategies to protect the health of the community, and ignore the importance of individual responsibility to act for the protection of others when a slavish adherence to rights of the individual puts others at risk of harm (Black 1992).

In light of such objections, no discussion of privacy can proceed without some preliminary account of its meaning and moral importance. A definition of privacy is discussed, as well as the underlying interests that make it morally significant, and how those interests are related to privacy rights is analyzed.

The second section applies the analytical framework to a discussion of how genetic information ought to be dealt with in the development of public policy. The importance of three distinct kinds of privacy rights is debated: Two rights described as rights of informational self-determination reflect the individual's interest in controlling, first, what information is generated and, second, what information is disclosed to others. A third kind of privacy right makes no reference to any liberty right or right of control vested in the individual. Instead, it is presented as a right against the government for protection against the loss of privacy, and it is of primary importance when privacy protection through the exercise of individual control over information is ineffective, infeasible, or undesirable. Finally, it is argued that what often matters most is that social and economic institutions are organized in ways that reduce the harmful consequences of increased access to personal information.

Privacy: A Framework for Moral Analysis

Privacy Definitions

Some privacy definitions are too broad for our purposes, such as the one frequently attributed to Samuel Warren and Louis Brandeis. Their view of privacy is often described as the right to be let alone (Warren and Brandeis 1890). However, as critics have noted, there are many ways of failing to let someone alone (e.g., hitting someone with a baseball bat), and most do not involve a loss of privacy (Thomson 1984).

Other privacy theorists have defined privacy as a condition of limited access to some aspect of the person (Allen 1987). A loss of privacy is said to occur when there is increased access to some aspect of the person. The specific kind of privacy loss individuals experience will depend upon the particular aspect of the person made more accessible. For example, limited access definitions might count as a privacy loss any one or more of the following aspects of the person for which access is gained: personal information (informational privacy); the person's body (physical privacy); the physical proximity of the person (solitude or seclusion) (Gavison 1984); a person's relationships with others (relational privacy); or a person's sphere of decision-making (decisional privacy) (Tribe 1978).

Multidimensional privacy definitions, or ones that count inaccessibility to more than one aspect of a person as forms of privacy, are the subject of considerable debate (Schoeman 1984). However, this chapter focuses primarily on informational privacy. Informational privacy can be understood as a condition or state of affairs in which access to information about a person's physical and mental condition, biological and genetic makeup, psychological states, dispositions, habits, and activities is limited.

Several implications of this definition, as well as some additional assumptions about the value of privacy, should be noted at the outset. First, privacy is always a matter of degree, and concern with its protection must always be tempered by the knowledge that it is not possible to ensure complete privacy.

Second, privacy merely describes a state of affairs; it is morally neutral. Privacy or its loss may be viewed as good, bad, or a matter of indifference. Its moral importance, if there is any, lies elsewhere. Thus, privacy is not assumed to be a fundamental category of moral thought. Its value is derivative from the underlying interests that may be promoted or protected when a condition of limited access to information exists.

Third, to the extent that privacy matters morally, what matters most in some instances is a certain kind of desired outcome, namely that access to information is restricted. It is an outcome that is desirable, independent of whether it is achieved by the individual's retaining control over personal information. In other instances, what matters most is that the individual retain and exercise control over access to information, even if doing so results in greater privacy losses than otherwise would occur under different social arrangements.

Fourth, the proposed definition of privacy comprehends limited access to information, not only by others, but by oneself as well. Thus, privacy losses include instances in which the individual gains access to previously unknown information about himself or herself.

Fifth, a loss of privacy is a morally significant event only when there is a reasonable expectation that access to information about a person will remain restricted.

Underlying Interests

What considerations form the basis of a reasonable expectation that access to personal information should be limited? This question takes on added urgency if privacy is not seen as a fundamental category of moral thought and if its value is viewed as wholly derivative of some underlying interests. One prominent approach to answering this question seeks to identify the *one* interest that explains why privacy matters in all instances (Reiman 1976). A number of possibilities have been suggested by various privacy theorists.

First, a person's well-being, or life prospects, may depend on limiting others' access to certain information, which if revealed can have adverse psychological, social, or economic consequences. Second, the ability to make personal choices without substantial interference by others may be compromised by access to information by those who may unduly influence personal decisions (Benn 1971). Third, access to information about a person may inhibit his or her ability to form intimate relationships with others where a selective sharing of information is often an essential element of what distinguishes deep personal commitments from the variety of other personal relations people share (Fried 1968). Fourth, intrusions into decisions about what information individuals will have access to have the power to affect profoundly personal self-concepts and the capacity for maintaining a sense of psychic stability (Reiman 1976). Fifth, dissemination of highly sensitive personal information may result in emotional distress, social stigma, embarrassment, and loss of self-esteem and the respect of others.

However significant any one interest may be in a wide range of cases, there is no compelling rationale for supposing that the moral significance of privacy in all instances is reducible to one underlying justification. A more plausible hypothesis is that there is not just one, but many interests that may matter morally; and often it is a cluster or constellation of interests that justifies concern for privacy protection.

Consideration of the importance of privacy in the context of genetics adds support to the cluster theory of privacy interests. Access to genetic information has the potential to adversely affect each of the interests identified above; in many instances, access to such information can create risks to social, psychological, and economic well-being, as well as threats to the exercise of autonomy and to the development of personal relationships.

The Nature of Genetic Information

The focus upon the cluster of interests at stake directs attention to the following questions: Is the information obtained from genetic testing and screening qualitatively different from other medical information? Is there anything about the nature of genetic information, or its potential uses, that makes it more deserving of privacy protection than other kinds of medical information? Several differentiating characteristics of genetic information have often been noted.

1. Genetics can reveal much more personal information about an individual than other types of medical testing and evaluation.

2. Genetic testing offers the often unwelcome prospect of revealing to individuals detailed predictions of their medical futures.

3. Genetic disorders generally affect people throughout their lives, and thus knowledge of genetic information may have a greater impact upon individuals than knowledge of other kinds of medical information.

4. The development of genetic information has potentially serious adverse financial, emotional, and social consequences.

5. The analysis of DNA samples may reveal information in the future not contemplated at the time of initial consent for testing or sample collection.

6. Genetic information has the potential to be misleading or incorrect in particular cases, in that it often relies upon probabilities for whole populations, whereas other personal and environmental factors can influence health outcomes.

7. Genetic testing or research into familial patterns of genetic inheritance may reveal information about other family members as well as information about a single individual.

None of these claims is sufficient to distinguish genetic information from a variety of other medical information routinely gathered. Many other medical tests and routine medical histories reveal much about other family members and about an individual's probable medical future. Information gathered from sources other than genetics may have adverse social and economic consequences, and it may be misleading or false. Other medical tests may reveal conditions that might affect persons throughout their lives, and future researchers and practitioners may learn things about the subject or patient not contemplated at the time of the initial encounter.

All these concerns taken together, however, illuminate the larger set of concerns attendant to the growth of scientific knowledge, of which genetics is but one very conspicuous reminder. What seems to magnify concerns about individual privacy is the increased potential for comprehensive, systematic, and efficient collection of an abundance of medical information about a person. Accordingly, concern for the privacy of genetic information should be enhanced, even if there is nothing clearly unique about this particular form of medical information.

The Foundation of Privacy Rights

The discussion so far has proceeded in terms of an inquiry into the interests that give informational privacy in general, and the privacy of genetic information in particular, its moral significance. However, debates about privacy typically are cast in terms of privacy rights, and indeed, one rhetorical function of rights language is the way it highlights the need for enhanced privacy protection. Thus, the connection between a cluster of morally significant interests and privacy rights—apart from the rhetorical one—needs specification.

First, if the moral significance of privacy depends upon the cluster of underlying interests at stake, then the moral significance of those interests in a particular context will depend upon the kinds of harms threatened by a loss of privacy. Those harms will depend upon a variety of factors, including the vulnerabilities of persons under any given set of economic and social arrangements, the existence of prejudice and impediments to an individual's ability to establish relationships with others within one's community, and the cultural traditions and customs that shape the individual's sense of dignity and self-worth.

Second, rights need not be seen as unconditional; they represent generalizations about the kinds of interests that are of such importance as to justify the imposition of certain duties on others (Raz 1986). However, current privacy rights and the duties they entail, in any particular context, are a function of the contingent character of a person's interests, the specific threats to those interests, the available alternatives for their protection, and the extent to which each alternative addresses the full range of interests at stake.

Third, although the particular kinds of informational privacy that might be important to protect will vary, the persistent fact of human vulnerability will ensure a continuing value for privacy. However, to the extent that scientific, technological, and cultural developments transform the context in which human vulnerabilities exist, then the kinds of information that ought to be protected from access will change, as well as the kinds of protection needed.

Fourth, a commitment to privacy rights does not entail a commitment to absolute rights. In many instances, there is simply no reasonable expectation that access to some information should be limited; and even where there is a reasonable expectation of limited access, there may be countervailing reasons favoring disclosure. The task is to determine when the position that Alan Westin calls in this book privacy fundamentalism should be adopted and when the position he calls privacy pragmatism should be embraced (Westin 1993). The former view represents a strong commitment to privacy protection at the expense of other social goals, while the latter is more willing to make trade-offs on a case-by-case basis.

A morally acceptable public policy with respect to genetic privacy will be a mixed strategy or one in which elements of both the fundamentalist and the pragmatist view are incorporated, depending on the particular balance of competing interests at stake. In some instances, the privacy fundamentalist position should be adopted, and accordingly, the existence of stringent rights to informational privacy must be recognized. Although there may be relatively few instances in which individuals have a reasonable expectation of exercising an absolute veto over what information about them is made available to themselves or others, the point of discussing informational privacy in terms of rights is a more modest one. It is the claim that informational privacy reflects the existence of a variety of morally significant interests of such importance that any proposed intrusion must overcome a substantial threshold presumption against it for it to be justified.

The Application of Privacy Rights to Genetic Information

Rights of Informational Self-Determination

One interest often at the root of concern for protecting the privacy of genetic information is autonomy, or the ability of individuals to control their own destinies. Rights associated with autonomy interests are classified as liberty rights, or the rights of individuals to make their own choices and decisions substantially free from the interference of others. In the context of genetic information, such liberty rights include the right of the individual to control access to highly personal information. In large part, the importance of retaining control over information reflects a deeper concern for the protection of more general autonomy interests. For example, rights of informational self-determination are especially valuable when a loss of control over information can result in a loss of ability or freedom to make other important life choices.

Autonomy interests provide the principal foundation for two rights that can be understood as species of what a German court has labeled the "right of informational self-determination" (Flaherty 1989). Such rights may be exercised in either of two ways. Individuals may assert their rights to control what information is collected or generated, or they may exercise rights to control aspects of further disclosures of information, including the purposes of further disclosures and the identities of the recipients of information.

Control Over What Information Is Generated

Some rights of informational self-determination are based upon the assumption that as autonomous agents, individuals are entitled to decide for themselves (at least to some extent) what they, or others, may know about them. However, rights to control the uses of information, or to control the identities of its recipients, may not be adequate to ensure autonomy. In some instances, the only (or most) effective way to secure the individual's ability to make important life decisions free from the undue interference of others is through the exercise of control over the initial production or creation of some kinds of information.

One illustration of the importance of the right to exercise control over the generation of genetic information involves calculations of social and economic risks. In some instances, individuals can plausibly claim that they want to weigh for themselves a variety of medical and nonmedical risks against medical and other benefits of knowing information about their genetic makeup. As long as there are substantial risks of social stigma or potential loss of insurance or employment, and no available medical intervention once test results are known, it is not unreasonable that an individual may rationally conclude that the benefits of testing and the information it produces do not outweigh the risks that might flow from unwanted or improper disclosure (Faden et al. 1991).

Additionally, a right of control over what information gets generated has implications for the moral duties of those who collect and store genetic information. Adequate respect for individual autonomy and the right of informational self-determination make it incumbent upon health professionals to discuss the economic and social risks of unwanted disclosure and to present an accurate and realistic account of the legal and other privacy protections as an integral part of the process of obtaining informed consent for testing (Powers 1991).

A second risk individuals arguably would want to weigh for themselves is that, with further scientific developments, the predictive information generated might turn out to be incorrect. Announcement of the discovery of some new genetic marker is an increasingly common occurrence, but some of the reports that purport to identify genes responsible for certain predispositions to disease may turn out to be false or misleading. One risk is that there may be a short-term scientific consensus on some markers for genetic predisposition that may, after great harm is done to those tested and labeled, turn out to be not well founded. The risks of false labeling include unjustified discrimination in employment or insurance, emotional distress, or pressure to undertake ill-advised actions pursuant to medical recommendations for risk reduction, e.g., prophylactic mastectomies or hysterectomies designed to reduce cancer risks. These are matters that ought reasonably be left for individuals to weigh against the claimed benefits of testing.

A third set of examples includes what is often called a right not to know (Shaw 1987). The emphasis of informational privacy is on ensuring that certain information is not made available to those the individual does not want to have access. This can include oneself as well as others. It is a right of privacy because it is one of the most important aspects of the person for which there is a reasonable expectation of limited access. The reasonableness of this expectation is supported by its close connection with what any conception of what autonomy minimally requires, together with considerations of the extreme sensitivity of certain types of information, and the potential for such information to produce profound psychological harm or interference with the exercise of autonomy.

Such considerations point to the kinds of risks one should reasonably expect to weigh in the decision about what information gets generated. The frequently discussed example of Huntington's disease is illustrative. Each individual may want to weigh for himself or herself the benefits of knowledge, which may aid in planning for the future, against the psychological burdens of emotional distress, chronic anxiety, and anticipation of development of a debilitating late onset condition.

Other examples highlight the close connection between risk of error and the potential for severe adverse psychological consequences. One example involves the sensitivity of certain tests, such as those used in carrier screening. If there is a substantial risk that couples identified as at-risk through population screening may be falsely labeled, there is the potential for needlessly increased levels of anxiety and for unwarranted interference with reproductive plans. Similarly, the risk of psychological harm from learning information about genetic predisposition to disease—which may never develop or may occur with only moderate severity—is the kind of risk that ought to be left to individuals to weigh for themselves.

The Generation of Information in Research Contexts

There are other instances in which arguments for a strong right of informational self-determination appear less well supported. Special problems of privacy protection arise in the context of pedigree studies generated from genetic registries. Such registries are designed to enable researchers to learn more about the natural history of that condition and the patterns of genetic inheritance. Patients identified as having symptoms or presymptomatic genetic predisposition for an autosomal dominant disorder (e.g., Huntington's disease, polycystic kidney disease, etc.) may be recruited for participation in a genetic registry. Each participant provides a detailed medical and family history, including the names of others in the family who may be affected by, or are at risk for, the disorder. Researchers use this information to develop a pedigree plot, which permits them to study the patterns of inheritance within a family. Family histories, as well as individual medical histories and perhaps even certain demographic information, are generally included in such registries.

Although the primary source for identifying persons to be included in a registry may be through referral by health care providers, and their inclusion in the registry comes only after informed consent has been obtained, a registry is likely to contain information about numerous other members of families in which the disorder has been prevalent. Typically, an individual gives consent for inclusion of his or her own name and history in the registry, as well as the names of and pertinent data about other family members. Thus, important information regarding nonparticipants is generated without the opportunity for nonparticipants to refuse.

Should nonparticipants be given the absolute right of control over what information is generated in this context? An answer depends upon a number of considerations. First, if the inclusion of nonparticipants poses a substantial risk of their learning of their own at-risk status or of learning that they are affected, then the case for a right to control what information is generated would be strengthened. In most of these cases, however, this is a minimally important consideration. Such persons are likely to have some awareness of their at-risk status as a result of their experiences with other family members. For example, with autosomal dominant conditions both sexes inherit the disease with equal frequency, and at-risk offspring of an affected individual have a 50 percent chance of inheriting the disease. In such cases, it seems unlikely that many individuals will be put at risk of learning new and unwanted information about their own conditions or risks.

Moreover, unless the confidentiality protections of the registry are especially poorly designed, there is a comparatively small risk of either the nonparticipant or others gaining access to information that could cause psychological, social, or economic harm. Researchers can take a variety of steps to ensure privacy that result in considerably less risk of adverse consequences of unwanted disclosure than with medical information in ordinary medical records. First, they should refuse to release data to participants regarding other family members without the latter's permission.

Second, researchers should segregate the data collected in the registry from all patient care records so that no individual will be adversely affected in insurance or employment by virtue of its inclusion in records accessible to employers and insurers. Any data obtained from the registry should be incorporated into medical records only with informed consent of the person who may be affected by possible disclosures.

Third, such registries should be protected from access by those having unrelated purposes. This can be achieved through the process of obtaining a Certificate of Confidentiality for research supported by the Public Health Service (PHS) as well as for nonfederally funded research related to alcohol abuse and alcoholism, drug abuse, mental health, and other health research. (1) The effect would be to shield such information from access by others, including law enforcement officers who might assert a need to know for purposes other than research. The certificate is not currently available for research not directly supported by the PHS, but the protection it affords should be extended to cover it.

If such safeguards are adopted, then the argument for a right of nonparticipants to control what information is generated is weakened considerably. In research contexts having adequate safeguards in place, there are reasonably persuasive arguments for thinking that the privacy pragmatist position is better justified than the privacy fundamentalist view.

However, the substantial costs of building a wall of separation between research activities and institutions delivering medical services must be acknowledged. The costs are justified in striking a reasonable balance between the need to conduct valuable scientific research for the common good and the needs for individual privacy protection.

Control Over Disclosures

The second form of the right of informational self-determination is related to the interest in controlling further disclosures. The right presupposes that information has been generated and that once it is generated and revealed to designated persons for specific purposes, individuals have a continuing interest in controlling what happens to it. This is an important element of privacy and confidentiality protection notably absent from most laws on medical information (Powers 1991). Control over the identity of the recipient, the purposes for which the information is used, and the period of time within which future disclosures may be made is too often lost once an initial consent to disclosure is given.

One illustration of these kinds of concerns in the genetic context involves the use of DNA databanks and databases. Although most scientific researchers ordinarily think of DNA banks established in conjunction with specific genetic registries, such as the Huntington's Disease Research Roster and DNA Data Bank at Indiana University, there is no established definition of what counts as a DNA bank. Databanks may be established for commercial, military, law enforcement, or a variety of other purposes. Even something as simple as the storage of a relatively small number of blood samples could have the potential for great harm if no procedures are in place to ensure privacy protection. Some current repositories of blood samples collected in conjunction with specific newborn screening programs (e.g., Guthrie cards) could become the basis for establishing databanks for new and previously unimagined purposes. In short, any collection of blood samples on filter paper—if well preserved, capable of being linked to identifiable persons, and organized in a searchable manner—can be transformed into a data bank with an enormous impact on privacy. The important point about the vagueness of the notion of a databank is that any repository of genetic information, regardless of the purposes for which DNA material was initially obtained, can be an attractive source for mining information for other purposes.

Nonetheless, the most troubling issues are raised by certain kinds of DNA databanks. Unlike academic databanks established for specific scientific purposes, some large-scale databanks can be far more comprehensive in the information they might contain, less well defined in their purposes and objectives, and developed on a mass scale.

One statewide plan to take blood samples of convicted felons illustrates the problems of databanks created for purposes other than research (de Gorgey 1990). For all persons convicted of felonies, a blood sample is taken and labeled with a numeric code. In a second file are personal identifiers and personal information including prison medical examination information, sentencing reports, etc. A third file consists of a barcode, or digitalized equivalent of the actual blood sample. In a fourth file is an integrated database containing all the barcodes. However, in most instances where someone submits to particular medical tests, that person may anticipate that a particular bit of information will be obtained and that it will reveal information of an anticipated sort for which consent for testing has been given. But storage of DNA information in blood samples—and perhaps barcodes, depending upon what is included—provides a ready source for discovering new information about which the individual did not give consent and which may not have been possible to anticipate. Those in possession of DNA samples have the ability to ascertain further information that vastly outstrips the scope of the purposes which provided the initial justification for collection.

If the right of informational self-determination is to be taken seriously, one public policy option would be to require specific consent for every contemplated redisclosure not comprehended in the initial plan. Although there are strong arguments to be made against *any* implementation of databanks in prisons and the military, at minimum, the individual should have the right to control the subsequent release of information for new purposes.

Disclosure Issues in Research Contexts

Although it has been argued that multipurpose and large-scale databanks are likely to pose the greatest threats to privacy, there are some additional privacy issues that emerge in research databanks. For example, academic genetic databanks are an attractive resource for others who assert a need to know for reasons unrelated to research, such as law enforcement. However, such arguments should be resisted. The ready access to medical and research data by law enforcement officials involves an unacceptable blurring of institutional roles and purposes. Health care providers and researchers should not be expected to bear the burdens of effectuating other arguably important social goals, however great those needs may be. To demand that health care and medical researchers assume the functions of law enforcement agencies compromises the ability of health care and medical research institutions to fulfill their primary missions. Without a social agreement that recognizes the need for a moral division of labor among its institutions, important social institutions cannot be expected to maintain the integrity and independence necessary to function effectively.

However, the justification for limiting further access for other health-related purposes is less compelling. Particularly vexing is the issue of how to strike a balance between the needs of epidemiologists and the needs of subjects for privacy protections. The controversy over the appropriateness of individualized consent for access to personal data for epidemiological research has been especially acute in European countries where members of the European Data Protection Commission have issued a draft report, already ratified by some countries. The draft report prevents access to and processing of data revealing ethnic or racial origin and data concerning health or sexual life without express written consent of each person about whom information is obtained. Critics argue that such directives will "legislate epidemiology right out of existence" (Editorial 1992). The concern is that such absolute rights of informational self-determination would prevent transmission of individual data to regional cancer registries, exclude use of data from persons who are dead or untraceable, and make retrospective studies of health records impossible (Knox 1992). Even if some of these complaints are overstated, it seems more reasonable to prefer privacy protection measures that are less disruptive of scientific advancement than individualized and explicit consent requirements.

Consider once again the rights of privacy in the context of pedigree studies. The position that individuals should exercise an absolute veto over their inclusion in such registries, subject to the important qualification that stringent privacy protections be in place, has been argued. In part, this argument was premised on the claim that these registries and databanks are distinguishable from the more general kinds of databanks we have just considered. In the nonresearch databanks, individuals are less likely to be adequately protected from unwanted disclosures. Additionally, genetic registries differ in the limited purposes for which they are created, in the kinds of protection that can be expected from exercise of rigorous review by Institutional Review Boards, in the use of Certificates of Confidentiality that can shield them from inquiries for unrelated purposes, and, one hopes, by the special sensitivities to the particular kinds of privacy risks associated with specific heritable disorders for which the registry was created.

Even if research and nonresearch registries and databanks differ in the ways previously described, there are some circumstances in which subjects should have the right to exercise some control over subsequent disclosures to other researchers. At minimum, participants should have the benefit of an informed consent procedure that adequately informs them of the kinds of risks posed by disclosures to other researchers and by the subsequent publication of their findings. Moreover, it would seem reasonable to require explicit consent for disclosures to researchers when the new uses of information exceed or differ from the purpose for which original consent was given. It would be presumptuous to assume that consent to disclosure for some research purposes is sufficient for all research purposes, especially in light of the fact that future research may focus on different conditions or genetic predispositions.

In most cases of epidemiological research not involving the release of the names of the persons, the risk of harm from disclosures to other researchers is small. However, the distinction between participants and nonparticipants in genetic registries is relevant. If nonparticipants have no right to veto inclusion of data regarding their conditions, then there is a need to ensure that institutional privacy protections are extended to external researchers who have access to identifiable data. When the names of those in the registry are shared with others, additional risks of unwanted disclosure are greatly increased. Before data are provided to someone not under direct institutional supervision and control, members of the Institutional Review Board need to approve a comprehensive and detailed privacy protection plan. No less stringent safeguards can be justified when nonparticipants are involved.

Pedigree Studies and the Protection of Anonymity

When the data are themselves the pedigree plot of the family, publication becomes problematic (Powers 1993). The risk is that publication of such data may result in inferential identification of individual family members. The risk of inferential identification may be increased when the publication of data reflects the geographic region from which the subjects were recruited or when the data describe a comparatively rare disorder.

One approach to the problem would be to require specific consent to the publication of pedigree data. Each family member would have the opportunity to personally review the proposed material in order to evaluate the likelihood of unwanted inferential identification. By contrast, an argument for a more pragmatic approach is that studies that are based upon incomplete family pedigrees, i.e., where individuals can prevent inclusion in the registry, undermine the scientific usefulness of pedigree studies. However, the fact that the publication of such data can potentially reveal the identity of nonparticipants who have not given informed consent (and who may not have had the opportunity to prevent the inclusion of their name in the registry) supplies a strong counterargument in support of the more stringent approach.

One can look for additional guidance on this question by examining the standards for protecting against inferential identification when the data reported in journals are photographs or case reports. The Statement from the International Committee of Medical Journal Editors offers some insight to the prevailing norms in these contexts (International Committee 1991). In the case of photographs, masking (e.g., covering a subject's face) may be adequate to prevent physical identification. Case reports are more problematic. They provide a richer, more detailed body of data that increases the possibility of inferential identification of specific persons. Where substantial risk to anonymity remains, the guidelines encourage specific informed consent as well as a clear statement in the article that such consent was obtained. The reasoning appears especially relevant to issues surrounding publication of pedigree studies. Pedigree studies can further compromise anonymity in that the base of information from which inferences may be drawn often is larger and the number of persons potentially affected is greater. By extension, it would seem appropriate to expect application of the same standard to the publication of pedigree studies. Hence, in spite of the practical problems of obtaining informed consent, it seems reasonable and consistent with established privacy norms among medical journal editors and researchers to start with a strong presumption in favor of informed specific consent from all potentially affected parties.

Particular attention should be given to the following considerations in any decision whether or not to publish. First, there are differences in the probability of inferential discovery. The greater the probability of loss of anonymity, the more important individual consent becomes. Second, there are differences in magnitude of expected harms. For example, some matters may be especially sensitive, and the expected magnitude of harm will be greater. These would include studies of families with a high prevalence of psychiatric conditions such as bipolar affective disorder. Third, there are differences in expected social benefit. Where the contribution to the growth of scientific knowledge is substantial, the case for publication even without explicit consent is strengthened. Fourth, the foreseeability of false labeling or having unaffected family members perceived by others as at greater than actual risk or affected by the disorder is especially important when stigma and prejudice are associated with certain conditions. Fifth, cases for which there is no informed consent to inclusion in a registry or, more importantly, where some have explicitly refused to participate, increase the threshold presumption against publication of the data in their complete form.

What alternatives are available if risks of inferential identification are significant and the prospects of obtaining informed consent from all the family members are poor? Two obvious possibilities exist. First, the decision might be made to scramble or disguise the data, such as by deleting a branch of the family tree or by altering birth order or gender. However, to the extent data are materially altered, this would be an unacceptable research practice, not only for reasons of scientific integrity, but because it undermines the risk—benefit calculus essential to the initial decision whether to publish. The undermining of the scientific validity and the ability of others to evaluate and replicate results destroys the expected benefit that provides a rationale for publication in the first place (Riis and Nylenna 1991). A second alternative is to publish results using some representative or hypothetical pedigree, coupled with the retention of the raw data by the journal under safeguards designed to limit inspection to bona fide researchers. Such suggestions present a variety of logistic difficulties, but the search for a new approach to communication with professional peers would be preferable to publication in the original form.

Information Disclosed for the Protection of Others

The issue of disclosure of genetic information to third parties in order to protect them from harm is one of the most complex issues to be addressed. Numerous persons have some claim of a legitimate need to know genetic information about particular persons for their own protection. Spouses and other reproductive partners may assert a need to know information that would affect reproductive decision-making (Wertz and Fletcher 1991). Fellow employees and unions may assert a need to know information that is relevant to assessing shared occupational risks and to protecting coworkers (Andrews 1991). Employers and consumers of services may seek information relevant to assessing fitness and suitability to perform certain kinds of jobs, such as whether airline pilots are likely to suffer the debilitating effects of diminished motor skills and judgment in the early stages of Huntington's disease.

However, not all potential interests that may be adversely affected justify disclosure of genetic information. The judicial system has not resolved these questions, and it is somewhat premature to predict the outcome of such cases (Robertson 1992). The recommendations of the President's Commission for the Study of Ethical Problems in Medicine and Biomedical and Behavioral Research (1983) are relevant both to the ethical and legal analyses of these issues. The authors of the report argue that patient confidentiality may be overridden when the following four conditions are met:

1. Reasonable efforts to elicit voluntary consent to disclosure have failed;

2. There is a high probability that harm will occur if the information is withheld, and the disclosed information will actually be used to avert harm;

3. The harm that would result to identifiable individuals would be serious; and

4. Appropriate precautions are taken to ensure that only the genetic information needed for diagnosis and/or treatment of the disease in question is disclosed.

There are several important questions to be considered in the application of those criteria to the genetic context. For example, how does one compare the risks of harm associated with failure to disclose genetic information with the risks associated with the failure to disclose psychiatric information to third parties in imminent danger of physical harm, or risks associated with the failure to disclose HIV status to sexual partners of infected patients? How do we analyze the conflict in cases such as those in which a person with the diagnosis of Huntington's disease refuses to disclose the diagnosis to relatives at risk of developing the disorder or of passing it on to their children? How is the future prospect of disability handled, as in the example of the airline pilot? Are the obligations of medical researchers different from those of medical practitioners (Applebaum and Rosenbaum 1989)? Are the obligations of medical researchers and health care practitioners to particular people (such as spouses) more stringent than their obligations to the public at large? How important is it that the harm that would result is to identifiable individuals as opposed to the public at large, as in the airline pilot case?

In most instances, those who are potentially harmed by lack of genetic information are not personally at risk in quite the same way as in the cases of psychiatric and HIV disclosure. One may not be convinced that the model used in these instances is appropriate in the genetic context. Additional questions might include the following: Are there further steps that others could reasonably take in the genetic context to avoid potential harms to the next generation, including initiation of alternative forms of testing for themselves? Is there the same immediacy of harm that only disclosure by physicians and researchers could foreseeably prevent? Moreover, apart from the harm to the next generation, often there is nothing that can be done to avert harm to existing relatives, and even if so, it is important to consider whether they could take steps for their own protection. Is it likely in cases such as that of the airline pilot that current procedures for detecting disability and fitness to perform such a demanding and responsible job are inadequate to protect the public such that the responsibility for doing so justifiably falls upon health professionals?

Until questions of these sorts are resolved, it is advisable to proceed cautiously with the extension of legal duties to protect in the genetics area, especially with extension to researchers who are not involved with patient care and counseling. In addition, the further moral importance in preserving the trust and privacy of the physician—patient relationship is of such importance that we should not rush to extend exceptions to the usual rule of confidentiality to these newer contexts, absent a compelling demonstration that the prevention of harm could not be achieved in a less intrusive manner.

When Control Is Not What Matters Most

There are some circumstances in which an individual has an interest in information being inaccessible to others or perhaps even to oneself; but in such circumstances, that interest may not be well served by means of individual control over access to information. The point is not that the efforts of others to protect privacy can be an adequate substitute for the privacy protection that one might otherwise achieve for oneself though one's own control. The point is that, in some instances, it is preferable that others act on one's behalf. The existence of such circumstances suggests that, in addition to liberty rights, there are cases in which the promotion and protection of an individual's privacy interests justify the existence of rights to be protected by others against certain harms. Two types of examples are illustrative.

First, individual control is not sufficient for protection against genetic privacy losses when genetic testing of one person reveals information about another. There are a number of examples of this phenomenon. Carrier screening for cystic fibrosis (CF) reveals information about the status of siblings as potential CF carriers. The use of genetic linkage studies in Huntington's disease produces results for other family members.

The heart of the problem is that the mere liberty right of each individual to exercise control over his or her own genetic information may not be sufficient for privacy protection when genetic information about one person can be obtained by third parties from another person. Hence, the privacy of each individual simply cannot be assured through a system of individual liberty rights where each exercises control over his or her own information; hence, the family member's dilemma.

What are the potential solutions to the family member's dilemma? One possibility would be to view the rights of control as collective rights, or ones vested in groups rather than in individuals. One could prohibit any testing of one person unless all others potentially implicated by such tests consented. The result would be a system of privacy protection that would prevent access by third parties in a way that a scheme of individual rights would not.

Although the performance of some genetic tests requires at least some cooperation by some other family members, the collective rights approach has severe drawbacks. One is the obvious problem of delineating the domain of all those affected by a decision to be tested (or to participate in linkage or pedigree studies). A more significant problem is that it would unreasonably deprive some persons of valuable benefits that may be derived from testing. Persons tested for CF could use the information obtained to make important reproductive decisions, and persons tested for susceptibility to Huntington's disease could make use of the information obtained for the development of other significant life plans. It would seem difficult to justify the denial of such benefits to one family member in order to preserve the privacy of another family member.

An alternative involves a right of the individual to be protected from third party (e.g., employer and insurer) access to information about one individual *via* access to a relative's medical file or other health data record. In short, the rationally preferred strategy would be a system of rights, which includes rights that those who are in a superior position to secure privacy protection act on the behalf of those who cannot protect their own interests through their own choices and actions. In most cases, these rights will be rights against the government for the kinds of protection that neither the individual nor nongovernmental entities are able to guarantee.

A second example in which individual control over genetic information is not sufficient to protect privacy focuses on another inadequacy of a liberty rights approach. In these cases, individuals would rationally prefer some sort of mandated restriction prohibiting their own disclosure of genetic information. The result would be that they could not voluntarily relinquish their own rights to privacy, i.e., the Ulysses strategy. Like the mythical figure from which its name derives, it may be rational to make present choices that have the result of relinquishing one's freedom to make choices in the future (Elster 1979).

The rationale for adopting Ulysses's strategy can be seen in the context of a market for health insurance. A system of liberty rights that vests in each individual the freedom to decide what information is given to insurers or employers may be an inadequate approach to privacy protection. When individuals lack equality of bargaining power, and the consequence of failure to disclose genetic information is an inability to obtain insurance or employment, then it is rational to prefer institutional restrictions that eliminate the liberty of personal control over such information.

Although the examples, in which privacy protection without control over information matters most, may be few in number, they are nonetheless among the most significant elements of a comprehensive genetic privacy protection strategy. Such rights to have one's privacy interests protected by others (typically by government regulation) reflect the limits of a liberty rights approach to privacy. Developments in genetics reveal contexts in which reliance on individual informational control is either impossible or rationally undesirable.

The Mitigation of Adverse Consequences

A paradoxical feature of rights is that it may be more rational to prefer a system with fewer rights to a system with more rights. This paradox is a consequence of the fact that rights have their moral importance in the face of threats to individual interests. Thus, the elimination of the conditions that threaten those interests makes a system of rights less important. The paradox of rights has important implications for arguments about the need for privacy rights in genetics. Many of the motivations for seeking greater privacy protections are predicated upon assumptions about the nature of the threats to our interests under a particular set of social and economic arrangements. However, it may be preferable to modify existing institutional arrangements in order to mitigate the adverse consequences that flow from unwanted disclosures.

Among the most important consequences of privacy losses in contemporary American society are economic ones, such as the loss of insurability. For example, insurers (and self-insured employers) might have fewer incentives to gain access to personal information if reforms in the market for health insurance were enacted into law. If the costs and eligibility requirements for health insurance were no longer dependent upon individual medical status or on the risk-based characteristics of a pool of insureds, then one important source of privacy concerns would diminish. However, it must be noted that any attempt to mitigate privacy concerns through the elimination of adverse consequences of disclosures raises fundamental questions of distributive justice in an explicit way. Any discussion of the relative weight of privacy in competition with other individual interests and social goals implicitly involves some view of just distribution. Consideration of policy options designed to make the need for privacy protection less pressing simply makes it clear that discussions of privacy rights cannot be pried apart from the hard questions of distributive justice.

Policy Implications and Conclusions

Reflection on the need for privacy protections in the context of the proliferation of genetic information raises some additional policy questions: Should there be special policies and laws for confidentiality and privacy protection with respect to genetic information? Or can existing laws governing medical information be relied on?

There are three reasons to think a separate genetic information policy, by itself, would be inadequate. First, to the extent that genetic testing becomes integrated into routine medical practice, the information will become a part of all medical records and thus open to the wide audiences to which medical records are now available. Second, because blood samples from any medical context can yield DNA information, there are serious difficulties with any proposal that attempts to define a databank and to specially regulate it separate and apart from the rest of medical practice. Third, to the extent feasible, public policy should leave it to individuals themselves to decide what kinds of information they are most concerned about keeping private and confidential. Thus, laws are needed that are adequate for the protection of medical and health-related information generally, and one should be reluctant to presume what kinds of information are most important to different persons.

Even if some special rules are desirable for pedigree studies and genetic databanks, the likelihood that genetic information will be increasingly incorporated into routine medical records suggests the need to review the adequacy of present medical privacy protections generally. Although a comprehensive assessment is beyond the scope of this discussion, there are three primary problem areas that should be mentioned (Powers 1991).

First, there are problems of regulation. Current laws contain numerous gaps. There are simply too many individuals and institutions that are not under a clear legal duty to maintain confidentiality. Moreover, even for those under a clear legal duty to protect confidentiality, too often they may be required to disclose information to a large number of persons and institutions for a wide variety of reasons having nothing directly to do with the delivery of patient care.

Second are problems of legal remedy. There are numerous impediments to effective civil suits for breach of privacy. Often breaches occur without the knowledge of those affected. Lawsuits are costly, both in financial and emotional terms. Lawsuits may be counterproductive inasmuch as the substance of the original grievance is the fact that highly personal or sensitive information has been revealed without one's permission and damage has thereby been caused, but the successful prosecution of a civil case requires the further airing of that information in an open public forum. Criminal prosecution may be even less effective. Successful criminal prosecution requires a higher burden of proof than civil trials, and in some instances victims may encounter prosecutorial reluctance to pursue powerful individuals and institutions. Discrimination suits designed to compensate for adverse consequences associated with unwanted disclosure may be ineffective for many of the same reasons that civil suits for breach of confidentiality are problematic. They present similar proof problems, particularly when intent is an issue in the case. Moreover, they may not offer an effective deterrent, especially if potential benefits of largely undetected discrimination outweigh risks of a few successful lawsuits.

Third are problems of jurisdiction. Medical information is collected, stored, and analyzed in a variety of states with different laws. A consent to medical tests in one state (under its laws) provides no assurance that similar legal protections will be available in other states where the information ultimately reaches.

Most current policies for privacy and confidentiality protection are designed to deter improper disclosures and to provide compensation for adverse consequences when the laws have failed to deter. The privacy interests outlined suggest a need for very different kinds of public policy options than the ones traditionally recognized in American law. There is a need for greater individual control over the generation and flow of information in some instances, for greater restrictions on the sharing of information than the currently accepted doctrines of a bona fide need to know now recognize, and for the elimination of certain predictable adverse consequences of information dissemination.

The challenges to personal privacy posed by the advances in genetic knowledge offer a welcome opportunity to rethink public policies with respect to medical and other health-related information in general.

Acknowledgments

Additional support for this research has been provided by the University of California, Los Alamos National Laboratory, Contract # 5–LJ2–7741E. Comments on earlier versions of this chapter were provided by L. Andrews, J. Childress, M. Frankel, S. Puck, K. Quaid, J. Robertson, and D. Runkle. Responsibility for errors and confusions remains my own.

Notes

1. Under Section 301 (d) of the PHS Act, a Certificate of Confidentiality may be applied for through the following agencies: for alcohol abuse and alcoholism research, contact the National Institute on Alcohol Abuse and Alcoholism, 14–C–20 Parklawn Building, 5600 Fishers Lane, Rockville, MD 20857; for drug abuse research, contact the National Institute on Drug Abuse, 10–42 Parklawn Building (same address as above); for mental health research, contact the National Institute of Mental Health, 9–97 Parklawn Building; and for all other areas of health research, contact the Office of Health Planning and Evaluation, PHS, 740G Humphrey Building, U.S. Department of Health and Human Services, Washington, DC 20201.

References

Allen, A. 1987. *Uneasy Access: Privacy for Women in A Free Society.* Totowa, NJ: Rowman and Allenheld.

Andrews, L. 1991. "Confidentiality of Genetic Information in the Workplace." *American Journal of Law and Medicine* 17:75–108.

Applebaum, P. and Rosenbaum, A. 1989. "Tarasoff and the Researcher: Does the Duty to Protect Apply in the Research Setting?" *American Psychologist* 44:885–94.

Benn, S. 1971. "Privacy, Freedom, and Respect for Persons." In J. Pennock and J. Chapman, eds., *Nomos XIII: Privacy*. New York: Atherton Press.

Black, D. 1992. "Personal Health Records." *Journal of Medical Ethics* 18:5–6.

de Gorgey, A. 1990. "The Advent of DNA Databanks: Implications for Informational Privacy." *American Journal of Law and Medicine* 16:381–398.

Editorial. 1992. "Protecting Individuals; Preserving Data." *Lancet* 339:3.

Elster, J. 1979. *Ulysses and the Sirens*. Cambridge: Cambridge University Press.

Faden, R., Geller, G., and Powers, M. 1991. "HIV Infection, Pregnant Women, and Newborns: A Policy Proposal for Information and Testing." In R. Faden, G. Geller, and M. Powers, eds., *AIDS, Women and the Next Generation*. New York: Oxford University Press.

Flaherty, D.H. 1989. *Protecting Privacy in Surveillance Societies*. Chapel Hill: The University of North Carolina Press.

Fried, C. 1968. "Privacy: A Rational Context." *Yale Law Journal* 77:475–493.

Gavison, R. 1984. "Privacy and the Limits of Law." In F. Schoeman, ed., *Philosophical Dimensions of Privacy*. Cambridge: Cambridge University Press.

International Committee of Medical Journal Editors. 1991. "Statement From the International Committee of Medical Journal Editors." *Journal of the American Medical Association* 265:2697–2698.

Knox, E.J. 1992. "Confidential Medical Records and Epidemiological Research: Wrongheaded European Directive on the Way." *British Medical Journal* 304:727–728.

Parent, W.A. 1983. "Recent Work on the Concept of Privacy." *American Philosophical Quarterly* 20:343.

Powers, M. 1993. "Publication-Related Risks to Privacy: The Ethical Implications of Pedigree Studies." *IRB: A Review of Human Subjects Research*. [forthcoming].

Powers, M. 1991. "Legal Protections of Confidential Medical Information and the Need for Anti-Discrimination Laws." In R. Faden, G. Geller, and M. Powers, eds., *AIDS, Women and the Next Generation*, 221–255. New York: Oxford University Press.

President's Commission for the Study of Ethical Problems in Medicine and Biomedical and Behavioral Research. 1983. *Screening and Counseling for Genetic Conditions*. Washington, DC: The Commission.

Raz, J. 1986. *The Morality of Freedom*. Oxford: Oxford University Press.

Reiman, J. 1976. "Privacy, Intimacy, and Personhood." *Philosophy and Public Affairs* 6:26–44.

Riis, P. and Nylenna, M. 1991. "Patients Have a Right to Anonymity in Medical Publication." *Journal of the American Medical Association* 265:2720.

Robertson, J. 1992. "Legal Issues in Genetic Testing." In American Association for the Advancement of Science, *The Genome, Ethics and the Law: Issues in Genetic Testing*, 79–110. AAAS Publication No. 92–115. Washington, DC: American Association for the Advancement of Science.

Schoeman, F. 1984. "Privacy: Philosophical Dimensions of the Literature." In F. Schoeman, ed., *Philosophical Dimensions of Privacy: An Anthology*. Cambridge: Cambridge University Press.

Shaw, M. 1987. "Testing for Huntington's Disease: A Right to Know, A Right Not to Know, or a Duty to Know?" *American Journal of Medical Genetics* 26:243–246.

Thomson, J. 1984. "The Right to Privacy." In F. Schoeman, ed., *Philosophical Dimensions of Privacy: An Anthology*. New York: Cambridge University Press.

Tribe, L. 1978. *American Constitutional Law*. Mineola, NY: Foundation Press.

Warren, S. and Brandeis, L. 1990. "The Right to Privacy." *Harvard Law Review* 4:193–220.

Wertz, D. and Fletcher, J. 1991. "Privacy and Disclosure in Medical Genetics Examined in an Ethics of Care." *Bioethics* 5:212–232.

PART III

Linking Genetics, Behavior, and Responsibility

INTRODUCTION

Genetic and Environmental Influences on Behavior

Alan I. Leshner, Ph.D.

The rapid recent growth of scientific knowledge about the role of genetic factors in health and in behavior, in combination with the immense promise of the Human Genome Project, stimulates both awe and concern in many lay and scientific observers. One can readily envision how increased knowledge and control of genetic factors can prevent illness, pain, and premature death and improve the quality of life. But past experience has shown us that an immense potential for harm can also be unleashed if genetic theories and data are misapplied and abused.

Nowhere is that ambivalent potential more evident than in the realm of behavioral genetics, where difficult scientific and social issues abound. Here, one must confront research questions concerning, for example, the nature of intelligence or mental illnesses; the variation of these traits within and across diverse populations; the relative contributions of heredity and environment to these variations; and the specific biological mechanisms that transmit and express genetic potentialities as behavior.

Answers to these questions are being pursued vigorously, but the causal chains are intrinsically complex and difficult to elucidate. To the best of current knowledge, most human behavioral traits of interest are not under the control of single genes, and most are likely to be influenced at least as heavily by environmental factors as by genetic factors. As V. Elving Anderson reminds us in the chapter presented here, a large fraction of the genome is devoted to the brain—"half of our 50,000 or more genes can be considered 'brain specific.'" But "genes do not directly *cause* behavior. . . ." In fact, it is hard to believe that behaviors will ever be discovered—beyond those that are reflexive—that are completely under genetic control. And to add to the scientific complexity, while genes certainly influence behavior, behavior can also influence genes.

Despite striking research progress in the past decade, one cannot yet reliably predict, prevent, or treat problem behaviors on the basis of genetic information about individuals. However, a time is approaching when, for better and for worse, individuals may be able to determine genetic vulnerability to certain classes of behavioral traits or genetic predispositions to respond in certain ways to particular types of environmental circumstances.

And so, while we seek to clarify the link between genetics and behavior, we must also seek to understand and address the many social implications of such research and its applications. This latter task requires special sophistication and clarity of thought to retain balance at the dizzying intersection of science, philosophy/theology, and law.

The four chapters presented in this section meet this challenge well, although in diverse ways. All make it clear, however, that scientific research—and particularly scientific research related to human behavior—is inextricably embedded within a complex web of social values. Indeed, it informs and is informed by those values. Both sides of that reciprocal relationship are examined in these pages, although the impact of behavioral genetics on the value sphere—particularly our views of individual responsibility or "agency" (and the related concept of free will)—is a major focal point.

Taken together, these chapters help to map boundaries of concern about an undeniably controversial aspect of scientific research and point to a number of issues that need further exploration. These include

1. The nature of multiple gene influences and what this means in understanding "causation" of behavior

2. The legal, ethical, and clinical implications of there being both social and genetic vulnerabilities for problem behavior and their expression in actual behavior

3. The responsibility and capability of scientists and clinicians to prevent/avert inappropriate interpretations and applications of behavioral genetics research and

4. The legal and ethical difficulties (including consent issues and stigmatization) of conducting behavioral genetics research with normal, at-risk, and problem-affected populations

As knowledge of potential gene-environment influences on behavior grows, these issues will need explicit attention.

5

Genes, Behavior, and Responsibility: Research Perspectives

V. Elving Anderson, Ph.D.

The Human Genome Project has social, ethical, and legal implications for a wide range of medical conditions. Relatively little attention, however, has been given to its possible impact on understanding human behavior. Yet behavioral problems are important, since they may affect perceptions of self and others and may alter views of moral and legal responsibility. In this context, two questions should be considered:

1. Are the implications of the Human Genome Project for behavioral traits different (in kind or in degree) from those for other problems?

2. What safeguards are needed in studies of behavior with respect to the design and interpretation of research, the welfare of individuals and families, and the relevant social and legal policies?

Pathways Between Genes and Behavior

First, some popular misunderstandings must be corrected. As Duster (1990) has pointed out, "There is a tendency to confuse heredity with inevitability and destiny, and to adopt a fatalistic stance." To be sure, there are rare circumstances in which a gene has such a strong effect that it appears to determine one's destiny. The same may be said for environmental events that can swamp genetic potential. Few, if any, behaviors are completely without genetic influence, and few behaviors are completely without environmental influence.

Genes do not directly *cause* behavior, since their effect is expressed indirectly through physiological systems. Furthermore, genes do not *determine* one's destiny in a predictable manner. The pathways are complex and are affected by experience throughout development.

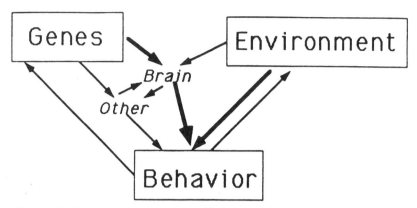

Figure 1. Pathways between genes and behavior.

A major link between genes and behavior (Figure 1) is the brain, which is the most complex and highly organized organ of the body. What is not generally realized, however, is that half of our 50,000 or more genes can be considered "brain specific" (Bloom 1989). Why such a large fraction of the genome is devoted to the brain is still a matter of conjecture. Furthermore, the expression of these genes varies over time (developmental age) and space (specific areas of the brain). If brain development were controlled by a computer, a part of the program would be devoted to organizing and scheduling the rest of the database.

Gene expression in organs other than the brain also can affect behavior. Phenylketonuria (PKU), for example, involves a liver enzyme that secondarily affects the brain. Adrenal steroids have important effects on brain function. Albino mice have lower activity scores than pigmented mice when they are tested under white light. However, this difference largely disappears when tested under red light, indicating the role of sensory input. More general features, such as physique and health, may also be important.

Furthermore, the pathway between genes and behavior is not unidirectional. Genes may indeed influence certain behaviors, but behaviors may also affect genes. Seizures, for example, can induce abnormal patterns of selective expression of a class of genes known as "immediate early." These genes, in turn, may play a critical role in long-term synaptic plasticity. Hormones released under stress also can change the relative expression of a number of genes.

It has long been realized that environment is a significant part of the picture. For purposes of analysis, the environment may be divided into internal, physical, biological, and psychosocial components. Furthermore, individuals are not merely passive recipients of external forces, since they may select and modify their environments. This element of choice is implied in the term *responsibility*, which is part of the title for this chapter.

Finally, the interplay among these several components changes as the organism develops. Each step is affected by the life experience up to that time. Thus, the development is not rigorously preprogrammed but is responsive to events as they occur.

The analysis of this complex pattern can be approached either by studies of the brain or by the evaluation of behavior. (It has been more difficult to identify trait-relevant aspects of the environment.) It is appropriate to start with the brain, however, because the immediate products of genes can be identified first at that level. Later on, the necessarily more indirect studies of behavior can be discussed.

Genes and the Brain

"The brain will be to the next century what the gene has been to the 20th century. . . . But compared to the gene, the brain . . . seems an infinitely more daunting objective" (Watson 1991, xv).

The laboratory of Craig Venter (formerly at NIH and now in private industry) has identified thousands of gene segments ("sequence-tagged sites") that are actively expressed in the brain. The functions of the tagged genes are unknown, but later they can be traced to specific chromosome locations and used as markers for gene-mapping studies, or more direct methods for determining the gene products may be devised.

Gregor Sutcliffe and Floyd Bloom (1989) chose a different strategy to reduce the enormous numbers of gene products to the smaller numbers that appear to be "interesting" for a specific investigation. They focused on the primate neocortex and began to identify the different kinds of messenger RNA (mRNA) that are expressed in the visual cortex, the motor cortex, and the prefrontal cortex. This several-step technique permits the identification of those mRNAs that are produced at much higher levels in one of these brain areas than elsewhere.

The important point here is to ask how such a massive amount of new information will be used in the future. One clue to the answer comes from the very complex and intricate steps involved as the mature brain develops from the simpler neural tube.

Development of the Brain

An overview of the complexity of brain development can be seen in Dominick Purpura's "recipe" for building a brain (pers. comm. 1992):

1. Take 200 billion neurons and a trillion glial cells. (Neurogenesis)

2. Mix with 100 neurotransmitters and modulators. (Chemogenesis)

107

3. Add two dozen growth factors and hormones. (Trophigenesis)

4. Arrange neurons in 500 sets, distribute nonrandomly. (Migration; Place specification)

5. Allow growth of dendrites and axons. (Neuronal differentiation)

6. Wire-up neurons each with many others in 10^{15} connections. (Synaptogenesis)

7. Eliminate redundant neurons and connections. (Programmed cell death)

8. Insulate rapidly conducting axons. (Myelination)

9. Use networks often and meaningfully. (Functional validation)

10. Do not abuse with toxins, trauma, or trivia.

Each of these steps involves the action of genes that are revealed by specific mutations. The pattern of formation, migration, and eventual fate of neurons resembles a symphony with several movements (Fischbach 1992; Kandel, Schwartz, and Jessell 1991). The early steps involve genes that lay out the basic segmentation of the primitive brain and genes for cell adhesion molecules. In the migration phase, the neurons follow cues, both structural and biochemical, which are partly under genetic control. The final differentiation of neurons into subtypes relies more on signals from the immediate environment surrounding the neurons.

Some areas generate too many neurons, and the extra ones are removed by genetically programmed cell death, which is a normal process. Excessive cell death may occur, as in Parkinsonism, and research is directed toward finding ways to retard the process. In cancer research, on the other hand, the goal is to find ways to induce selective cell death.

Cell-to-cell communication is made possible by chemical messengers (neurotransmitters) that interact with channels and receptors or by molecules that pass through gap junctions (pores on the cell surface formed by "connexins"). These mechanisms for neuronal signaling have been of considerable recent interest, and a number of genes have been identified that are relevant for studying behavioral variation. Consequently, this aspect of neuroscience is singled out for special attention in the following section.

Neuronal Signaling

A single nerve cell may receive connections from hundreds of neurons that use different chemical transmitters. This input to a single cell could not take place unless there were different kinds of receptors sensitive to the different transmitters. Some of these receptors contain distinct channels that open or close to control the flow of specific ions (calcium, sodium, potassium, or chloride), while others trigger biochemical changes within the cell. Thus the central neuron must integrate a diverse set of inputs into a coordinated response.

Excitatory synaptic action is mediated by receptor-channels that are selective for sodium and potassium. The major excitatory transmitter in the brain is glutamate. *Inhibitory* synaptic action is mediated by receptor-channels selective for chloride, and the major inhibitory transmitters are gamma-aminobutyric acid (GABA) and glycine. (These antagonistic forces, excitation and inhibition, provide a fine-tuning control of neuronal activity that has been likened to the balancing effect of accelerator and brake in a car.)

A sodium ion channel gene was first isolated and cloned from *Drosophila* (the fruit fly). The product of this single gene has 24 transmembrane domains that surround a central pore through which sodium ions can pass. The *Drosophila* gene has since been used to isolate sodium channel genes in the mouse and the human.

The receptors for GABA, glycine, and glutamate, on the other hand, are constructed by combining subunits that are produced by genes on different chromosomes. The situation is made more complex by the fact that there are three types of GABA receptors (A, B, and C) depending on their response to other substances in addition to GABA. The $GABA_A$ receptors are composed of at least three subunits (α, β, and γ) that differ in the strength of binding to GABA. Each subunit in turn has variations ($\alpha1$ to $\alpha6$; $\beta1$ to $\beta3$; $\gamma1$ and $\gamma2$) that are produced by different genes. The various combinations of subunits permit an amazing *receptor diversity*, which may increase the information-handling capacity of neurons. In some situations the "mix" can be altered in response to changes in the local environment, thus providing a major mechanism for brain plasticity.

As the brain matures, neurons in different parts of the brain switch on or switch off the expression of different GABA receptor subunits. These changes in receptor composition may be important for establishing inhibitory circuitry. Furthermore, a mutation in one gene in this gene family may have a noticeable effect only in certain parts of the brain at certain points of development or on certain types of functions.

A number of other receptors are also under genetic control. Dopamine receptors are primary targets for drugs used in the treatment of disorders such as Parkinson's disease and schizophrenia, and the genes have been cloned for six of them (D_1, D_{2a}, D_{2b}, D_3, D_4, and D_5). The D_4 receptors are of special interest since they bind clozapine, a drug that is unusually effective in treating schizophrenia, 10 times better than other dopamine receptors. Furthermore, the D_4 receptors are thus far the only dopamine receptors that show genetic variation (polymorphism) in human populations (Van Tol et al. 1992). This combination (population variation in a gene product with special interest for a behavior) is just what is needed to test the hypothesis that some individuals with schizophrenia may have a mutation in that gene.

Molecular Genetic Strategies

The availability of molecular methods has led to many new research options in the neurosciences. No longer is one limited to observation. The opportunities for intervention now permit a more direct test of hypotheses, and three general research strategies have been developed.

1. *Express a gene.* Once a specific gene has been identified, an expression vector containing the mRNA for that gene can be introduced into cells that can make the gene product. Ovary cells are well equipped with raw materials and enzymes to respond to fertilization by rapid growth, and this potential can be tapped for experimental purposes. For example, the genetic code for an ion channel protein, when introduced into a Chinese hamster ovary cell, permits the cell to make and deposit ion channels in the cell membrane. The functioning of the ion channel can now be tested in its new setting.

2. *Change or block expression of a gene.* By site-directed mutagenesis it is possible to change a gene in a specific manner. Thus, hypotheses about the structure of ion channels can be tested by altering small sequences of the channel gene in order to determine which parts are critical for a given function. Translation of messenger RNA can be blocked by inserting antisense RNA (a complementary mirror image that binds to the mRNA and blocks its further function). More recently, copies of an inactivated gene have been injected into cells with the result of an exchange for the normal gene and a "knock out" of its function (Travis 1992).

3. *Insert a new gene.* Finally, copies of a gene construct (a synthesized gene) can be introduced into cells and become incorporated into a chromosome without significantly altering the genes already there. In this way transgenic animals and transfected cell lines can be produced.

Studies of the Cerebellum

These new methods can be illustrated by reference to a specific brain area. The cerebellum has functional as well as structural features that make it particularly well suited for further genetic study. The mouse cerebellum, for example, is readily accessible and has a reasonably simple architecture. Furthermore, mutations affecting the mouse cerebellum result in obvious movement disorders and thus have been given graphic titles: *swaying, weaver, staggerer, reeler,* and *lurcher.* There are also a number of mutations in humans that lead to disorders of coordination (the ataxia), which result from neurophysiological disturbances of the cerebellum.

A specific mutant gene in the mouse, *Purkinje cell degeneration,* results in a 95 percent loss of Purkinje cells in the cerebellar cortex (similar to some human ataxias). In order to understand the effect of this degeneration, three transgenic mouse lines have been developed, carrying copies of a gene construct expressed only in Purkinje cells and causing their death (Feddersen et al. 1992). The results show that late cell death has little effect on the rest of the cerebellum, but early death causes a decrease in the migration and proliferation of granule cells and may also affect glial cell interactions. These, and other genetic manipulations, provide powerful techniques for exploring the effects of mutant or abnormally expressed genes on the developing structure and function of the brain.

Linking Neurogenetics With Behavior Genetics

The underlying goal for research in the genetics of behavior is to trace the pathway from a gene to events in the brain and thence to behavior, but research studies on the several steps in this pathway often are isolated and poorly interconnected. An excellent example of an effort to develop a more complete explanation can be found in the recent use of a "knock-out" mouse to study learning and memory (Barinaga 1992).

Previous studies had shown that repeated stimulation of cells in the hippocampus starts a chain of events. Initially, receptors on neuronal membranes are activated, leading to an influx of calcium. As a result, the neurons show a greater response to the next signal, an effect that can be prolonged for some time. This phenomenon, termed long-term potentiation (LTP), is thought to be the physiological basis for some aspects of learning and memory.

The linkage to behavior is seen in the observation that drugs that block these receptors also block LTP and impair spatial learning in mice. The reactions within the neurons involve enzymes known as kinases (which activate proteins by adding phosphate), but it was not clear which of the several kinases were critical. This question could be tested by using molecular genetics methods to "knock out" the gene for a specific kinase and then to examine the effects upon LTP and spatial learning.

Mutant mice that lacked the gene for α-calcium-calmodulin kinase II (CAM kinase) were developed. Studies of hippocampal slices showed that LTP was deficient, confirming the hypothesis at the neuronal level.

Other knock-out mice with the same mutation were examined for their ability to use spatial cues to find a platform in a round pool of opaque water. In a series of tests, the mutant mice took considerably longer to learn the task.

In a parallel report from the laboratory of Eric Kandel (Grant et al. 1992), mice with knock-out mutations in four tyrosine kinase genes were studied with reference to LTP (in hippocampal slices) and also spatial learning and memory (in the water tank test). One of the mutants (*fyn*) showed a deficiency in both areas, whereas the other three were normal. This report adds another mechanism that can link genetic mutations to changes in learning and memory.

These studies clearly show that single genetic changes can have a selective and significant effect on learning and memory. Furthermore, application to humans can be envisioned. When the CAM kinase and tyrosine kinase genes are mapped to specific mouse chromosomes, one can look for variation in homologous human genes that might be correlated with behavioral variation. The enzyme and its effects also can be studied in hippocampal slices from postmortem human brain in conditions associated with severe memory loss.

Implications of Neurogenetic Research

The rapid pace of neurogenetic research is impressive. Literally thousands of DNA segments expressed in the brain are being identified, although information about the function of the complete genes lags considerably. The ability to manipulate these genes provides powerful research tools. In the future, some of these techniques may become useful in the treatment of human disorders, but the main use at present is for the understanding of gene function and regulation.

There is a high level of variability in the genes themselves, in the timing of their expression, and in the way their products are combined to make a functional entity, such as a receptor. Discovery of the primary cause of disorders thus becomes more difficult, since the critical mutant gene may be detectable only in a small part of the brain or at a specific point in development. Furthermore, the "cause" of a disorder may be different in subgroups of the population, making accurate prediction of predisposition difficult. As with other medical problems, the number of false negatives and false positives may be sizable early in the research.

In summary, brain development is complex and dynamic, involving a continuing interaction between genes, the internal environment, and (indirectly) the external environment. The brain at some points and in some individuals may have a surprising plasticity for responding to challenge. But an awareness of the complexity should temper the interpretation of new findings.

Genes and Behavior

A complementary strategy starts with behavior and works back toward the brain and the genes. This research approach must be adapted to the fact that most behaviors appear to involve many genes, each with a small effect. Furthermore, nongenetic factors are likely to be involved.

A number of research steps are needed for complete genetic evaluation (McGue and Gottesman 1989). The interpretation of results concerning a particular behavior should be qualified if the analysis is incomplete.

1. *Definition of the phenotype.* Objective criteria must be stated explicitly so that the results of different studies can be compared. These same criteria can be used to analyze the frequency of the trait, by age and in a specified population. As Troy Duster (1990) has emphasized, inappropriate or inadequate definitions at the beginning of a study will seriously confound efforts to interpret research results.

2. *Evidence for genetics.* Familial resemblance may result from genetic factors, environmental influences, or from a combination of these. Information from intact nuclear families may not provide enough information to analyze the "mix" of these factors, so it is desirable to utilize twin studies and adoption studies as well.

3. *Mode of inheritance.* The family data are analyzed, often with the aid of computer programs, to determine which of the following hypotheses best fit the data: (a) a single gene with major effect; (b) a multifactorial model, which assumes a number of genes, each with a small and equal effect; or (c) a mixed model, a combination of a major gene with other genes of minor effect.

4. *Role of the environment.* At the outset, it can be assumed that both genetic endowment and environmental stimulation are essential for the development of behaviors. However, if the contribution of one of these components is not recognized, isolated analysis of the other may give misleading results. It should be noted that *experience* may be a better term than *environment* for describing nongenetic influences on behavior (Turkheimer and Gottesman 1991).

5. *Gene mapping.* Finding the chromosomal location for a specific gene provides confirmation of the genetic basis for a condition and suggests whether or not all families with a similar phenotype will have the same condition. This has proved to be quite difficult, however, for some important behavioral problems.

6. *Pathogenesis.* If a gene for a trait is mapped and sequenced, further studies are needed in order to determine the gene product, to find out

how the gene is regulated (when in development and where in the brain it is expressed), and to explore the interaction with other genes and with environmental factors in the pathogenesis of the condition. The distinction between *etiology* (which may be genetic) and *pathogenesis* (the other mechanisms leading from the basic etiology to the expressed phenotype) is well recognized for medical problems such as cystic fibrosis and applies also to behavioral traits. As Matt McGue (1989, 508) has stated, "The day has arrived when showing that some trait is under partial genetic or environmental control without accounting for, or hypothesizing about, the mechanism of that influence will simply not do."

Given the complex features of the brain (described earlier), it is not surprising that behavioral traits often appear multifactorial in nature. In such circumstances, mathematical models can be used to analyze family data and partition the observed variability, or phenotypic variance (V_P), into its components: genetic (V_G), shared environment (V_{SE}) that is common to relatives reared together, and nonshared environment (V_{NE}). The relationship between these components is expressed in the following formula:

$$V_P = V_G + V_{SE} + V_{NE}$$

The portion of phenotypic variance that is due to genetic factors is termed the "heritability". It is important to note that heritability for a behavioral trait *is neither constant nor immutable*, but only describes the situation in a population sample at a given time. Under different circumstances at a different time the heritability could be considerably different. Eric Turkheimer and Irving Gottesman (1991, 19) emphasize the importance of both points of view: "In some contexts, it is perfectly reasonable to ask how individuals in their natural environment come to vary as they do; in others, it is reasonable to ask how they might vary if the environment were to be altered radically."

Furthermore, some other features of the gene—environment relationship are not captured by heritability estimates (Plomin, DeFries, and McClearn 1990, 250-251). Genes and environment may display several types of *covariance*: (1) passive, in which a child who inherits genes that promote the development of some behavioral characteristic is also likely to be reared in an environment that fosters the development of that same trait; (2) evocative, in which a child's behavior elicits a response from a parent, teacher, or other caregiver that further alters the child's behavior; or (3) active, in which a child is not merely a passive recipient of external forces, but selects and modifies the environment. Finally, genetically different individuals may respond in different ways to the same environmental factors, a situation known as gene-environment *interaction.*

Traits that appear to fit the mixed model present a challenge to efforts at gene mapping, since it may be difficult to locate a gene with major effect that is modified by a multifactorial background. Statistical methods have recently been used to search for major gene effects in quantitative traits, such as the size of tomatoes. This approach has been adapted for behavioral genetic studies in what is known as the quantitative trait locus (QTL) method (Plomin 1990). It has been proposed to use this method to study a given trait in appropriate mouse lines, using a number of markers that have been mapped to individual chromosomes. If a major gene effect is detected from markers on a specific mouse chromosome, attention would be turned to markers on the human chromosome(s) that carry homologous genes. Those markers then could be used to study human behaviors that appear to resemble the behaviors in the mouse.

Finally, development is as important for human behavior as for the human brain, since later stages are conditioned by prior experience. Furthermore, there may be critical time windows during which specific genetic and environmental factors may be particularly influential. Turkheimer and Gottesman (1991) have described the usefulness of the concept of *reaction norm* to depict variation in a phenotype as a function of genotype and environment, and the concept of *canalization* to describe variation in the reaction norm over time. These ideas help one to visualize the observation that "individuals get stuck in diverging ruts as they age" (Turkheimer and Gottesman 1991, 20). Similarly, "If organisms seek out suitable experiences as they develop, and if genetic expression depends on prior experience, the correlation between genotype and environment will increase with development, with a concomitant increase in diversity" (21).

Selected Research Areas

The current status of research is summarized below for selected behavioral conditions. Some are being studied at the molecular level, while others are recognized primarily by their social impact, thus illustrating the range of implications for the Human Genome Project.

Fragile X Syndrome

The fragile X syndrome is probably the most frequent cause of mental retardation in males. Earlier it was diagnosed by a thinning or actual break of the X chromosome in special cytogenetic tests. More recent research has traced the problem to a DNA triplet (CCG), which can be repeated many times (Kremer et al. 1991). An increased number of copies is associated with more severe retardation and a tendency toward even more amplification. When a woman has 50 or more repeats, the chance of yet more repeats (and hence more retardation) in a child is sharply increased.

The discovery of the triplet repeat was a major advance, but screening, testing, and counseling still are difficult. The pathogenetic mechanism leading to the retardation is still unknown, and there is no effective treatment as yet. Furthermore, some of the carrier mothers may be somewhat retarded themselves, and counseling must be adjusted appropriately.

Huntington's Disease

Individuals with Huntington's disease (HD) develop progressive neurological and behavioral deterioration, usually in adult life, and the risk of suicide is increased. The risk to the offspring of an affected person approaches 50 percent by the end of life, but much of adult life may be lived with the apprehension and uncertainty that signs of HD may yet appear. The discovery in 1983 that the HD gene is located on the short arm of chromosome 4 permitted, in informative families, a shift from a 50–50 risk prediction to a 95 percent or 5 percent risk, depending on the results of DNA marker testing.

Finally, the misuse in Nazi Germany of genetic information about HD led to political decisions that some lives are not worth living, followed by compulsory sterilization and other serious abuses (Harper 1992). This historical background and concern about losing medical insurance has led some HD patients to worry about the consequences of unauthorized disclosure of computerized medical records.

The careful attention that has been given to testing and counseling in such circumstances provides helpful models for dealing with other behavioral problems (Tibben et al. 1993). The main reasons that at-risk individuals give for seeking DNA testing are a desire to gain better control over their future (pregnancy planning or employment) and worry about the implications for spouse and other relatives. Decisions also must be made about using the tests for minors or for prenatal diagnosis. In HD one encounters all the issues seen for other adult onset medical problems (such as adult onset diabetes or polycystic kidneys) plus the fact that early signs of HD may alter behavior and the capacity to cope with the progressive disease.

Recently the basic genetic problem in HD was shown to be a trinucleo-tide (CAG) repeat, somewhat like the situation found in the fragile X syndrome (Huntington's Disease Collaborative Research Group 1993). The normal population may have from 11 to 34 repeats, but in HD patients the range is from 42 to over 66 copies. The function of the gene affected by this repeat area is not yet known, and no clues for possible therapy are yet available. Furthermore, study of other families and populations will be needed before more accurate risk determination is possible.

Substance Abuse

A marijuana receptor gene in the rat has been cloned and sequenced and has been expressed in Chinese hamster ovary cells (Matsuda et al. 1990). Further studies of the receptor in this system showed that the relative potencies of various cannabinoids correlate highly with those of the psychoactive cannabinoids that produce a "high" in humans. Expression of this receptor occurs in the basal ganglia, cerebral cortex, and hippocampus, providing further evidence that this receptor protein is involved in the cannabinoid-induced effects on the central nervous system that are experienced by users of marijuana. The human receptor gene has now been mapped to the long arm of chromosome 6 (Hoehe et al. 1991) and may become a good candidate gene for mapping behavioral and other disorders.

Work is now in progress to determine if there is human individual variation in both the coding and the regulatory regions of this receptor gene. If such variation is found, it will be possible to study the function of the variants in ovary cells or similar systems. Mutants that differ in their responsiveness to cannabinoids or that may even render their individual carriers unresponsive to the psychoactive potency of marijuana may be found. This approach could be used to study individual variation in response to other psychoactive drugs and to examine any relationship to the drug-seeking behavior itself. It may also be possible to test experimental modifications of the drugs in a search for those variant molecules that retain reported useful medicinal properties while losing undesirable psychoactive effects.

Schizophrenia

Schizophrenia is one of the most carefully analyzed human behavioral traits, and the evidence for the role of genetic factors is robust and widely accepted (Gottesman 1991). For example, all subtypes of schizophrenia were observed (in various combinations) in the Genain quadruplets, a monozygotic set who arose from a single fertilized egg and carried the same genetic predispositions. There is much indirect evidence for dopamine receptor hypersensitivity. Drugs, e.g., amphetamine, that increase dopamine levels can cause a psychosis that resembles the paranoid subtype of schizophrenia. All subtypes of schizophrenia have been treated by drugs that block dopamine receptors.

Yet the possibility is left open that several gene loci (perhaps four to eight) might be involved. In recent years, several gene-mapping

117

studies suggested linkage of a susceptibility gene to chromosome 5, but further work, with more informative DNA markers and the onset of new illness in family members, sharply reduced the evidence (Pauls 1993). There may be genetic heterogeneity (different mutant genes in different families), or some of the presumed cases may result from nongenetic mechanisms. Another problem in linkage analysis is dual mating, with susceptibility genes coming in from both sides of the family.

There is clear evidence for the role of (unidentified) environmental factors, since the risk to the monozygotic (MZ) cotwin of a schizophrenic index case is 48 percent, leaving the other half unaffected. The risk for offspring of the unaffected MZ cotwin is the same as for offspring of the affected index case (17 percent), confirming the hypothesis that the unaffected cotwin must have carried the gene(s) for susceptibility (Gottesman and Bertelsen 1989).

If genetic linkage should become established in some families, the possibility of linkage heterogeneity and the role of nongenetic factors will make risk prediction difficult. It is unlikely that the situation will be as clear as that for Huntington's disease.

Alcoholism

Alcoholism in a first-degree relative is a robust predictor of risk for alcoholism. The trait is not easily identified in a given individual, however, and it is difficult to find control families without alcoholism. Twin and adoption studies have convincingly established the existence of genetic influences on the etiology of alcoholism in men, but the role in women remains largely unclarified. In men, the tendency toward early-onset alcoholism is more heritable than that for the late-onset form.

There have been extensive efforts to find genetic markers for alcoholism (McGue in press). Earlier it was thought that individual variation in dopamine D_2 receptors was an indicator of susceptibility, but it now appears that there is little relationship to alcoholism per se. (There are indeed large population differences in D_2 genes and in alcoholism, but the two factors are easily confounded.) There is better evidence for a genetic effect in Asians. A genetic deficiency (in one of the enzymes that metabolizes alcohol) is found in about half of the general population in China and Japan, but in only 12 percent of their alcoholics. Apparently the deficiency permits the accumulation of toxic intermediates, thus *reducing* the chance of developing alcoholism.

In mice and rats the intake of alcohol, the sensitivity and tolerance to alcohol, and the effects of alcohol withdrawal show evidence of genetic control. Long-sleep (LS) and short-sleep (SS) mouse lines, for example, have been selectively bred for high and low hypnotic sensitivity to a sedative dose of ethanol. The LS line is also more sensitive to other depressants. Further studies of these two lines have provided evidence that GABA pathways are involved. This is confirmed by studies in which the messenger RNA for GABA$_A$ receptor from the mouse brain was introduced into oocytes (Wafford et al. 1991). The effect of alcohol on GABA was seen only when a GABA receptor subunit gene has an extra segment of eight amino acids.

Omenn (1988, 579) has pointed to human alcoholism as "a worthy challenge for elucidating and modeling genetic and environmental interactions." He urged investigators to target specific phenomena including (1) predisposing personality, cognitive, neurophysiological, and cultural factors for drinking behaviors; (2) susceptibility to acute effects; (3) metabolism of ethanol; (4) central nervous system effects— tolerance, dependence, and addictability; and (5) susceptibility to medical and behavioral complications.

Intelligence

Normal cognitive ability must involve a very large number of genes and gene products that interact with factors in the internal and external environment. Yet a mutation in a single gene (or gene pair) can interfere dramatically with normal development. Severe retardation in a child often represents the effect of a single genetic or environmental change (such as a genetic error of metabolism or an intrauterine viral infection). Mild retardation, on the other hand, is usually the net effect of a number of factors, each with small effect and seldom detectable.

Family studies of IQ data permit three further generalizations (Turkheimer and Gottesman 1991): (1) there is a moderate linear relationship between parental genotype and offspring intelligence; (2) severely deprived environments produce a powerful effect; and (3) there are very small environmental effects in the range of environments provided by intact families.

There also are some interesting effects of age. When data on adolescents from several large studies are combined, the heritability for IQ is about 0.50, suggesting that about half of the variability is genetic (Chipuer, Rovine, and Plomin 1990). In the most recent analysis of IQ data for adults, however, the heritability rises to about 0.80 (McGue et al. 1993). Among adolescents there is a sizable component for the shared environment, but among adults this component drops out and that fraction of the heritability is added to the genetic portion.

The frequency distributions shown in Figure 2 may give some perspective to these calculations. In the general population, 95 percent of individuals have IQ scores between 70 and 130, mainly as a result of the way IQ tests are standardized. If one could select all individuals with their genetic potential set at the average for the population, the genetic

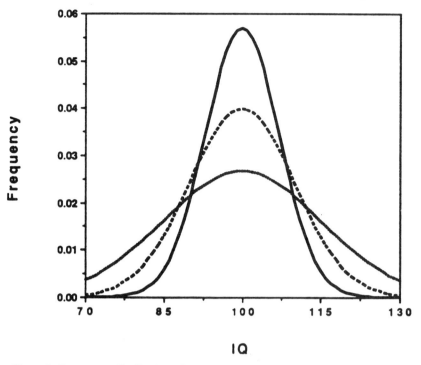

Figure 2. Frequency distribution of IQ scores. Individuals in general population (dotted line). Individuals with average genotype: Heritability = 0.50 (dashed line). Heritability = 0.80 (solid line).

variation would have been removed, leaving the variation resulting from environmental factors. If the heritability were 0.50, the 95-percent range in scores would be reduced somewhat, from 79 to 121. Even if the heritability were as high as 0.80, there would still be considerable variability in IQ scores, with 95 percent from 87 to 113. Thus, an individual's genetic potential may set a range of possibilities, but does not predetermine the results at a fixed point.

In some situations, genetic analysis has helped to challenge popularly held views. For example, the observation that children with lower school performance on the average come from larger families has led to a concern that the genetic basis for intelligence is declining. This interpretation, however, fails to take into account those who fail to reproduce at all. In one large study of (Caucasian) families, there was a negative correlation of parental IQ level with number of children, thus appearing to confirm the popular impression. When all siblings of the parents were included, however, the fertility was level across ability groups (Reed and Reed 1965). The conclusion was that the genetic basis for intellectual ability is stable and is not declining.

The interaction of race and socioeconomic status with intellectual performance was examined in data from 12 university medical centers as part of the Collaborative Perinatal Project (Nichols and Anderson 1973). In the sample from Boston, the socioeconomic index was relatively high but nearly identical for blacks and whites. In the combined samples from Baltimore and Philadelphia, the index was considerably lower as a result of clinic admission criteria but again was very much alike for blacks and whites. The mean four-year IQ scores, from individually administered Stanford-Binet tests, for white children from Boston were 15.4 points higher than the mean for black children from Baltimore and Philadelphia, similar to results from a number of other studies. Within each sample, however, the black—white difference was only four to six points. The conclusion was that socioeconomic factors are largely responsible for the usually reported black—white differences in intellectual performance.

Finally, in a more direct application of genetic markers made available through the Human Genome Project, Robert Plomin is analyzing the DNA from children who have been given a series of cognitive tests (Aldhous 1992). The goal is to identify alleles that are more common among children who score high on the tests and thus provide a clue to genes that may affect intelligence. Other samples will be studied in order to rule out chance associations.

Studies of this type in the long run may well contribute to understanding genetic factors involved in intellectual performance. However, random DNA markers that are found to be associated with cognitive tests results should not be used for *individual assessment or prediction* until the genes and gene products are identified and the underlying neural mechanisms are carefully explored (in order to establish the validity, and not merely the accuracy, of such tests).

Criminality

Criminality is not a simple trait for genetic analysis. Cases are sometimes obtained through official records in an effort to respect the privacy of individuals and also to collect a larger sample. The laws and administrative practices vary from one population to another, however, making comparisons between studies difficult. For some specific questions it may be better to use *antisocial personality disorder*, a recognized psychiatric diagnosis with defined criteria. One might alternatively attempt to measure an underlying personality trait, such as aggression or violence, but these are less well defined.

The XYY story illustrates some of the problems. The initial 1965 report, based on a prison sample, raised the possibility that XYY individuals are at high risk for violence and crime (Jacobs et al. 1965). A central concern in the controversy that followed shortly thereafter was that parental knowledge of the chromosome tests could become a self-fulfilling prophecy. As a result, ongoing studies were brought to a halt. Fortunately, there is more accurate information now from prospective studies that followed XYY children into adolescence (Carey in press). A summary of the results portrays them as a group of individuals within the normal range but with an array of relatively nonspecific behavioral differences in attention and cognition, motor skills, and personality. These problems may bring an individual to professional attention, but information about the XYY chromosomal status provides little, if any, guidance concerning care. The only criminal history is for minor offenses not characterized by violence and aggression.

More recently, in August 1992, another controversy developed (Palca 1992). NIH had approved a conference titled "Genetic Factors in Crime: Findings, Uses, and Implications." The list of invited speakers appeared reasonably well balanced, reflecting a wide range of points of view. A sentence in the advertising brochure, however, suggested options that are well beyond the current state of knowledge: "Genetic research holds out the prospect of identifying individuals who may be predisposed to certain kinds of criminal conduct, of isolating environmental features which trigger those predispositions, and of treating some predispositions with drugs and unintrusive therapies." A major controversy arose, stressing the racist potential in the general topic and in the proposed conference. In response, the NIH funding was withdrawn.

A few months thereafter, a report on violence was published from a panel of the National Research Council (NRC) (Reiss and Roth 1993). Among its summary findings was this more modest statement:

Strong evidence from Scandinavian studies points to genetic influences on antisocial personality disorder in adults, a diagnostic category that includes persistent assaultive behavior. Evidence of a genetic influence specific to violent behavior is mixed, however, and neither relationship has been studied in U.S. samples. If genetic predispositions to violence are discovered, they are likely to involve many genes and substantial environmental interaction rather than any simple genetic marker.

The NRC has commissioned a number of review papers that are to be published in several supplementary volumes. In one of these, Greg Carey (in press) has highlighted some tentative conclusions from genetic studies (of adoption in Denmark, Sweden, and the United States; of twins in Denmark and Norway; and of families in the United States) that may be useful in planning further analysis.

1. Genetic factors do not appear to be important in most cases of juvenile delinquency. The evidence supports a major role for home and sociocultural factors.

2. The contribution of alcohol abuse must not be minimized. In a Swedish adoption study, violent offenses by the biological father predicted the son's alcohol abuse better than the son's criminal record. Furthermore, crime associated with alcohol abuse was often against persons, whereas crime in the absence of alcohol abuse was nearly always against property only.

3. In both twin and adoption studies of adults, there was some evidence for genetic factors in the liability for crimes against persons and crimes against property, but there was no significant overlap between these two kinds of liability.

The NRC report and its supplementary volumes will provide an excellent basis for future research on this important, yet controversial, topic. A clearer consensus is needed, however, on reasonable expectations for the role of genetics in this complex and important kind of behavior. One guideline would be Gordon Trasler's (1987, 14) point that "if we are to make suggestions about the biological bases of criminality, we have to indicate what it is that is genetically transmitted—not simply that something exhibits a pattern of incidence that is consistent with familial transmission—and the essential stipulation is surely that whatever it is must clearly be relevant to the transactions between the individual and his social environment that issue in criminality or in conformity (or 'law abidance,' as Mednick calls it)." Finally, I agree fully with the comment by Robert Cloninger and Irving Gottesman (1987, 107) that "all attempts at intervention with high-risk families must be tempered by our limited ability to predict who will actually develop antisocial behavior and the imperative need to protect individual civil rights."

Related Issues

Reductionism and Responsibility

Neuroscience involves a reductionist effort to study the brain by tracing neural mechanisms back to cells and molecules. This powerful strategy often is the only effective way to approach important problems. There is a growing awareness, however, that this reductionism must be balanced by a "reconstructionism," which uses the new knowledge to frame an understanding of the brain with which the investigation started (Savageau 1991). The one approach is incomplete without the other.

Genetic analysis of the brain should utilize the research methods of both neuroscience and behavioral genetics. The effort to gain a more complete view, albeit more complex, is methodologically sound and will also reduce simplistic answers that may increase ethical problems. In a similar vein, Patricia Churchland (1986, 3) holds that "top-down strategies (as characteristic of philosophy, cognitive psychology, and artificial intelligence research) and bottom-up strategies (as characteristic of the neurosciences) for solving the mysteries of mind-brain function should not be pursued in icy isolation from one another. What is envisaged instead is a rich interanimation between the two, which can be expected to provoke a fruitful co-evolution of theories, models, and methods, where each informs, corrects, and inspires the other."

Gunther Stent's review of the history of molecular genetics provides an interesting historical perspective (1968). Research prior to 1953 had determined the physical and chemical *structure* of the DNA molecule, including its dimensions and the double helix conformation. The internal arrangement of the components in the form of the "DNA model" was not resolved, however, until Watson and Crick asked two fundamental biological questions dealing with *function*: How can DNA be copied faithfully? How can DNA carry information? The obvious lesson is that phenomena can be explained from the bottom up (in terms of physics and chemistry) so long as the questions are posed from the top down (from biology).

Now that explanations at the boundary between genetics and behavior are being considered, however, the possibility arises that success in explaining brain function might also "explain away" the basis for responsibility (see Cole-Turner's chapter). The "genes plus environment" equation seems to explain everything and leave no freedom for individual choice. It is already understood that everyone's personal freedom is shaped by genes and experience, although not all to the same degree or in the same way. How will new research change this perception?

The theoretical and philosophical problems have proved difficult to resolve, but identical twins provide a relevant experiment of nature. Although the similarities in behavior may be impressive, the cotwins are two separate persons. There does not appear to be any case in which one twin has effectively disclaimed moral or legal responsibility by pointing to the behavior of the other. Presumably, each would still be evaluated independently as a responsible person.

In this context, R. David Cole's (in preparation) view is welcome: "Our personhood emerges from the multi-dimensional interplay of our genes and our history of circumstances along with the present and past motivations of our spirit. Therefore, no matter how great the magnitude of genetic determinism, our sense of responsibility for who we are need not be overwhelmed."

Genetic Diversity and Human Equality

Some have claimed that the ethical principle of social justice provides the grounds for denying genetic diversity and resisting efforts to study it. The phrase "all men are created equal" in the Declaration of Independence has caused confusion and misunderstanding, since it seems to imply genetic uniformity. Fortunately, other early statements reflect a less ambiguous view of equality. For example, the Virginia Declaration of Rights (1776) held "that all men are by nature equally free and independent, and have certain inherent rights, of which, when they enter into a state of society, they cannot by any compact, deprive or divest their posterity." Thirteen years later, the French Declaration of Rights stated that "Men are born and remain free and equal in rights."

It is in this spirit that Theodosius Dobzhansky (1973) insisted that the recognition of genetic diversity should strengthen our resolve to promote human equality. Benno Müller-Hill (1993, 492) extended this view to say: "Laws are necessary to protect the genetically disadvantaged. Social justice has to recompense genetic injustice." They agree that we must recognize both diversity and equality.

Conclusions and Summary

Much of the recent discussion about the ethical implications of the Human Genome Project has been directed toward issues such as genetic testing in relation to insurance and the workplace, privacy and confidentiality of test results, and unfair genetic discrimination with reference to relatively rare single-gene medical disorders (Murray 1991; Robertson 1991). Genetic studies of human behavior can draw upon the recommendations from these reports, but major differences, at least in degree, arise from the fact that most behaviors are *biopsychosocial* in nature. The *origin* of behavior is conditioned by biological, psychological, and social factors, and the *identification* of "affected" individuals may be influenced by the social setting. Regimens prescribed for *intervention or treatment* often will include individual and group psychological measures in addition to medication. The net result is that behavioral phenotypes appear to be unique in the following ways, at least in their combined effect, and careful consideration is required to deal with their complexity.

1. *More persons in the normal range of functioning will be included.* Genetic research usually has been most rapid when applied to rare disorders. When the focus for study moves into the normal range, a multifactorial pattern generally emerges. Here, the criteria for a definition of behavioral variation will often become more subjective and, hence, potentially subject to manipulation by those who are creating and applying the labels or attempting to control the behaviors.

2. *Estimates of predisposition will be less precise.* When the range of variability in medical problems includes milder cases, many individuals with abnormal genotypes will be completely normal, falling into a category described as the "asymptomatic ill" (Billings et al. 1992). It is uncertain whether disability laws that cover discrimination in the workplace will protect those who are currently healthy but at genetic risk (McEwen and Reilly 1992). The situation is further complicated when we consider the fact that the accuracy of risk estimation declines rapidly as one goes from Huntington's disease to schizophrenia and then to alcoholism. If marker testing is proposed for addressing behavior, great care must be given to monitoring the accuracy of such tests and to defining the questions for which each test is valid.

3. *Environmental and experiential factors may play a larger role.* Behaviors generally involve a response to the environment, and they develop over time in response to the succession of experiences. This does not mean that all individuals are affected in the same way. McGue (in press) has emphasized the usefulness of a "diathesis-stress" model in which genetic factors contribute to individual differences in diathesis (predisposition). With low "genetic loading," only the most extreme environments can elicit the behavior under consideration, while with high loading the behavior develops readily in most environments. It is those in a middle range who are most sensitive to the relative intensity of environment stress. The mere invoking of "environment" in a general sense, however, is not enough, and research studies must look for specific elements of experience relevant to particular behaviors.

4. *A wider range of modalities for treatment or intervention will be used.* Discovery that a genetic factor contributes to development of a behavioral pattern does not mean that treatment at the genetic level will be possible or easy. Intervention may be safer or more effective farther along the pathway of pathogenesis and may involve a combination of medical and psychological methods. In particular, for behaviors that have been strongly influenced by experiential factors, it is likely that behavioral intervention may be needed. The goal will be to reduce identifiable barriers and to help each individual approach his or her own potential.

5. *There will be greater implications for individual freedom and responsibility.* The treatment of many medical problems often places a heavy reliance on the patient's compliance with respect to prescribed medications, but this becomes more problematic if the patient's behavior itself is affected by the medication. Medical geneticists do not now release genetic test data to insurance companies without consent; but it is not clear how this principle would be extended to similar requests

from a court or social agency that might limit the individual's personal freedom (imprisonment) or funding (welfare payments). Careful consideration of specific situations will be required since the fundamental ethical concern is to improve autonomy, in line with current efforts stressing personal responsibility for health.

6. *More professional groups will be involved.* The biopsychosocial nature of behaviors calls for a high level of interaction among professionals who may not be accustomed to such interchange. Some individuals trained in neurogenetics and behavior genetics may not be fully aware of the concerns that medical geneticists have for confidentiality of records and the vagaries of risk predictions. These three groups will need to become acquainted with the problems faced by teachers, therapists, social workers, and judges.

These comments are not intended to mean that research on genes and behavior should be prohibited. In the absence of relevant information, the actions of the general public and even of professionals may be guided by commonly accepted myths. Without the longitudinal studies of XYY males, for example, no one would have known that the effects are relatively mild. Furthermore, if the role of genetic mechanisms is completely disregarded, studies of presumed environmental factors may produce seriously misleading results.

The problem is with half-truth, the oversimplified result of inappropriate research design, or the public misunderstanding arising from premature release of tentative findings. The use of new techniques and data from the Human Genome Project in studies of human behavior should meet high standards in all stages of research design, implementation, and interpretation. Ethical considerations should include the subjects of investigation and their families (Shore et al. 1993), as well as the broader social setting, including the possibility of racism. The review of research proposals, for example, might include advocates for broader social concerns who could speak on behalf of an enlarged view of "informed consent." Finally, the ethical, legal, and social implications should be explored at all stages of research with judges, social workers, and other professionals who may become involved. The process will be complex and demanding, but the potential benefit for individuals and families may be great.

Acknowledgments

Helpful comments from participants at the Los Alamos conference and from the following are gratefully acknowledged, although responsibility for the opinions expressed remain with the author: D. Bartels, C.E. Anderson, X. Breakefield, J. DeFries, R. Feddersen, E. Gershon, D. Goldman, I. Gottesman, M. Hoehe, M. McGue, D. Murphy, H. Orr, J. Peterson, S. Rich, E. Ross, and J. Wehner.

References

Aldhous, P. 1992. "The Promise and Pitfalls of Molecular Genetics." *Science* 257:164–165.

Barinaga, M. 1992. "Knockouts Shed Light on Learning." *Science* 257:162–163.

Billings, P.R., Kohn, M.A., de Cuevas, M., Beckwith, J., Alper, J.S., and Natowicz, M.R. 1992. "Discrimination as a Consequence of Genetic Testing." *American Journal of Human Genetics* 50:476–482.

Bloom, F.E. 1989. "Strategies for Understanding the Role of Gene Defects in the Pathogenesis of Mental Disorders." In V. Bulyzhenkov, Y. Christen, and L. Prilipko, eds., *Genetic Approaches in the Prevention of Mental Disorders*, 45–56. Berlin: Springer-Verlag.

Carey, G. In press. *Genetics and Violence.*

Chipuer, H.M., Rovine, M.J., and Plomin, R. 1990. "LISREL Modeling: Genetic and Environmental Influences on IQ Revisited." *Intelligence* 14:11–29.

Churchland, P.S. 1986. *Neurophilosophy: Toward a Unified Science of the Mind/Brain.* Cambridge: MIT Press.

Cloninger, C.R. and Gottesman, I.I. 1987. "Genetic and Environmental Factors in Antisocial Behavior Disorders." In S.A. Mednick, T.E. Moffitt, and S.A. Stack, eds., *The Causes of Crime: New Biological Approaches*, 92–109. Cambridge: Cambridge University Press.

Cole, R.D. In preparation. *The Molecular Biology of Transcending the Gene.*

Dobzhansky, T. 1973. "Is Genetic Diversity Compatible With Human Equality?" *Social Biology* 20:280–288.

Duster, T. 1990. *Backdoor to Eugenics.* New York: Routledge.

Feddersen, R.M., Ehlenfeldt, R., Yunis, W.S., Clark, H.B., and Orr, H.T. 1992. "Disrupted Cerebellar Cortical Development and Progressive Degeneration of Purkinje Cells in SV40 T Antigen Transgenic Mice." *Neuron* 9:955–966.

Fischbach, G.D. 1992. "Mind and Brain." *Scientific American* 267:48–67.

Gottesman, I.I. 1991. *Schizophrenia Genesis: The Origins of Madness.* New York: W.H. Freeman.

Gottesman, I.I. and Bertelsen, A. 1989. "Confirming Unexpressed Genotypes for Schizophrenia: Risks in the Offspring of Fischer's Danish Identical and Fraternal Discordant Twins." *Arch General Psychiatry* 46:867–872.

Grant, S.G.N., O'Dell, T.J., Karl, K.A., Stein, P.L., Soriano, P., and Kandel, E.R. 1992. "Impaired Long-Term Potentiation, Spatial Learning, and Hippocampal Development in *Fyn* Mutant Mice." *Science* 258:1903–1910.

Harper, P.S. 1992. "Huntington Disease and the Abuse of Genetics." *American Journal of Human Genetics* 50:460–464.

Hoehe, M.R., Caenazzo, L., Martinez, M.M., Hsieh, W-T., Modi, W.S., Gershon, E.S., and Bonner, T.I. 1991. "Genetic and Physical Mapping of the Human Cannabinoid Receptor Gene to Chromosome 6q14-q15." *The New Biologist* 3:880–885.

Huntington's Disease Collaborative Research Group. 1993. "A Novel Gene Containing a Trinucleotide That Is Expanded and Unstable on Huntington's Disease Chromosomes." *Cell* 72:971–983.

Jacobs, P.A., Brunton, M., Melville, M.M., Brittain, R.P., and McClemont, W.F. 1965. "Aggressive Behavior, Mental Subnormality, and the XYY Male." *Nature* 208:1351–1352.

Kandel, E.R., Schwartz, J.H., and Jessell, T.M., eds. 1991. *Principles of Neural Science.* New York: Elsevier.

Kremer, E.J., Pritchard, M., Lynch, M., Yu, S., Holman, K., Baker, E., Warren, S.T., Schlessinger, D., Sutherland, G.R., and Richards, R.I. 1991. "Mapping of DNA Instability at the Fragile X to a Trinucleotide Repeat Sequence p(CCG) *n.*" *Science* 252:1711–1714.

Matsuda, L.A., Lolait, S.J., Brownstein, M.J., Young, A.C., and Bonner, T.I. 1990. "Structure of a Cannabinoid Receptor and Functional Expression of the Cloned cDNA." *Nature* 346:561–564.

McEwen, J.E. and Reilly, P.R. 1992. "State Legislative Efforts to Regulate Use and Potential Misuse of Genetic Information." *American Journal of Human Genetics* 51:637–647.

McGue, M. In press. *Genes, Environment and the Etiology of Alcoholism.* NIAAA Research Monograph Series. Washington, DC.

McGue, M. 1989. "Nature—Nurture and Intelligence." *Nature* 340:507–508.

McGue, M., Bouchard, T.J., Jr., Iacono, W.G., and Lykken, D.T. 1993. "Behavioral Genetics of General Cognitive Ability: A Life-Span Perspective." In R. Plomin and G.E. McClearn, eds., *Nature—Nurture in Psychology,* 59–76. Washington, DC: American Psychological Association Press.

McGue, M. and Gottesman, I.I. 1989. "Genetic Linkage in Schizophrenia: Perspectives From Genetic Epidemiology." In V. Bulyzhenkov, Y. Christen, and L. Prilipko, eds., *Genetic Approaches in the Prevention of Mental Disorders,* 24–38. Berlin: Springer-Verlag.

Müller-Hill, B. 1993. "The Shadow of Genetic Injustice." *Nature* 362:491–492.

Murray, T.H. 1991. "The Human Genome Project and Genetic Testing: Ethical Implications." In American Association for the Advancement of Science, *The Genome, Ethics, and the Law: Issues in Genetic Testing,* 49–78. AAAS Publication No. 92-115. Washington, DC: American Association for the Advancement of Science.

Nichols, P.L. and Anderson, V.E. 1973. "Intellectual Performance, Race, and Socioeconomic Status." *Social Biology* 20:367–374.

Omenn, G.S. 1988. "Genetic Investigations of Alcohol Metabolism and of Alcoholism." *American Journal of Human Genetics* 43:579–581.

Palca, J. 1992. "NIH Wrestles With Furor Over Conference." *Science* 257:739.

Pauls, D.L. 1993. "Behavioural Disorders: Lessons in Linkage." *Nature Genetics* 3:4–5.

Plomin, R. 1990. "The Role of Inheritance in Behavior." *Science* 248:183–188.

Plomin, R., DeFries, J.C., and McClearn, G.E., eds. 1990. *Behavioral Genetics: A Primer.* 2d ed. New York: W.H. Freeman.

Purpura, D. Personal communication, May 18, 1992.

Reed, E.W. and Reed, S.C. 1965. *Mental Retardation: A Family Study.* Philadelphia: W.B. Saunders.

Reiss, A.J., Jr. and Roth, J.A., eds. 1993. *Understanding and Preventing Violence.* Washington, DC: National Academy Press.

Robertson, J.A. 1991. "Legal Issues in Genetic Testing." In American Association for the Advancement of Science, *The Genome, Ethics, and the Law: Issues in Genetic Testing*, 79–110. AAAS Publication No. 92–115. Washington, DC: American Association for the Advancement of Science.

Savageau, M.A. 1991. "Reconstructionist Molecular Biology." *New Biologist* 3:190–197.

Shore, D., Berg, K., Wynne, D., and Folstein, M.F. 1993. "Legal and Ethical Issues in Psychiatric Genetic Research." *American Journal of Medical Genetics (Neuropsychiatric Genetics)* 48:17–21.

Stent, G. 1968. "That Was the Molecular Biology That Was." *Science* 160:390–395.

Tibben, A., Frets, P.G., van de Kamp, J.J.P., Niermeijer, M.F., Vegter-van der Vlis, M., Roos, R.A.C., van Ommen, G.-J.B., Duivenvoorden, H.J., and Verhage, F. 1993. "Presymptomatic DNA-Testing for Huntington Disease: Pretest Attitudes and Expectations of Applicants and Their Partners in the Dutch Program." *American Journal of Medical Genetics (Neuropsychiatric Genetics)* 48:10–16.

Trasler, G. 1987. "Some Cautions for the Biological Approach to Crime Causation." In S.A. Mednick, T.E. Moffitt, and S.A. Stack, *The Causes of Crime: New Biological Approaches*, 7–24. Cambridge: Cambridge University Press.

Travis, T. 1992. "Scoring a Technical Knockout in Mice." *Science* 256:1392.

Turkheimer, E. and Gottesman, I.I. 1991. "Individual Differences and the Canalization of Human Behavior." *Developmental Psychology* 27:18–22.

Van Tol, H.H.M., Wu, C.M., Guan, H.-C., Ohara, K., Bunzow, J.R., Civeill, O., Kennedy, J., Seeman, P., Niznik, H.B., and Jovanovic, V. 1992. "Multiple Dopamine D4 Receptor Variants in the Human Population." *Nature* 358:149–152.

Wafford, K.A., Burnett, D.M., Leidenheimer, N.J., Burt, D.R., Wang, J.B., Kofuji, P., Dunwiddie, T.V., Harris, R.A., and Sikela, J.M. 1991. "Ethanol Sensitivity of the $GABA_A$ Receptor Expressed in Xenopus Oocytes Requires 8 Amino Acids Contained in the γ2L Subunit." *Neuron* 7:27–33.

Watson, J.D. 1991. *The Brain.* Plainview, NY: Cold Spring Harbor Laboratory Press.

6

Human Genetics, Evolutionary Theory, and Social Stratification

Troy Duster, Ph.D.

Trouble at the Bottom, Virtue at the Top

From its very inception in the latter part of the nineteenth century, the science of human genetics germinated in, was nurtured by, and was inextricably entangled with the social and political storm of evolutionary theory. There has been both strong continuity and notable change with today's human genetic inquiry. Most commentators have chosen to emphasize the sharp differences with the past when it comes to the eugenic danger. For example, the esteemed historian of science Daniel Kevles has argued that, in today's society, vulnerable and marginalized groups have greater access to strategies and mechanisms for fending off any eugenic resurgence. There remains, however, a persistent search for "hard data," for a biological or biochemical explanation of homelessness, mental retardation and mental illness, alcoholism and drug abuse, even unemployment, crime, and violent and abusive behavior. The change has come in a thick disguise of the old concerns, the promise of untold health benefits and the lessening of human suffering. Some of these promises will be fulfilled, and some remarkable strides have already been made in the detection of genetic disorders.

Yet these successes have had an unwitting and inadvertent side effect. The demonstrable advances in biomedicine have produced a "halo" over a host of problematic claims about the connection between genes and behavior, so much so that we are witnessing the chameleon-like reincarnation of some of the more regressive formulations of late nineteenth-century thought.

On the surface, the Human Genome Project, a program to map and sequence the entire spectrum of human genes, has as its primary rationale the improvement of human health. The major strategy is the uncovering of genetic disorders and susceptibility to disorders and, ultimately, the hoped-for development of gene therapies to treat or cure those disorders (Kevles and Hood 1992; Proctor 1991a; Bishop and Waldholz 1990). But no matter how one slices it, just underneath the talk of a paradigmatic shift, society seems inexorably pulled back to the ancient concern for trying to explain what could be called "trouble at the bottom, virtue at the top," by reference to the properties of individuals.

From Biological Darwinism to Social Darwinism

One of the most enduring truths in the study of human social life is that all societies are stratified. The unequal access to valuable resources can be based on something as simple as age or as complex as claims to spiritual or intellectual power. But as far back as recorded history permits us to garner evidence, we also know that humans have always tried to justify that stratification. In *The Republic*, Plato creates the "myth of the metals" to justify why only those "born gold" can become philosopher kings. The notion that power and privilege are *inherited* has a longer and wider history than the notion that power and privilege are *achieved*. The link between a theory of human biology and social theory has always been a significant force in the history of ideas, but only in the last 150 years has the connection donned scientific clothing. At the core of this relatively recent development is the direct link between biological Darwinism and social Darwinism and the direct but underappreciated implications for the birth of human genetics. In order to appreciate the subtle, sometimes subterranean continuity between the past and the present, we must go back to those early beginnings.

Charles Darwin's *Origin of Species* is the bible of evolutionary theory, at once a meticulous classification system of organisms and a theory of the evolving relationships between them. In its simplest form, the implications of the taxonomy are known even to some grade-school children: at the bottom of the rung is the single-celled amoeba; at the top of the heap is the magnificently complex human. In between are all the combinations and permutations and mutations that form an intricate hierarchy of organisms. It is intricate. It is most decidedly a hierarchy. (1)

What of humans? Once we get to the top rung of the ladder of species evolution, biological Darwinism trails off and, like a relay sprinter in a race, huffing and puffing and tired, hands the baton to the runner in the next leg. The baton was passed from biological Darwinism to social Darwinism.

In the biological version of adaptation, species are ranked along a hierarchy of complexity in evolutionary adaptation, but what about rankings *within species?* Within, between, and among human groups, was there not also an evolutionary tree? As Darwin had done for biological Darwinism, the English social theorist Herbert Spencer (1820-1903) would issue the canon of social Darwinism. To better understand the climate in which scientific genetics germinated, it is necessary to rescue and restate two important features of late nineteenth-century thought that have been largely forgotten. The first is that Spencer dominated the social thought of his age as few have ever done. By far the most popular nonfiction writer of his era, his ideas were so popular that he sold over 400,000 copies of his books during his lifetime.(2) In the United States, by the turn of century Spencer attained the status of a dominant cultural figure among a wide range of American politicians, intellectuals, educators, and public policy advocates (Hofstadter 1955). Indeed, he was so influential that Oliver Wendell Holmes once sardonically turned to his colleagues on the Supreme Court to remind them that "Herbert Spencer did not write the U.S. Constitution" (Seagle 1946).(3)

Although Darwin would ultimately distance himself from the more regressive social implications of Spencer's social evolutionary theory, Darwin once called Spencer "about a dozen times my superior" (Darwin 1959, 2:239).(4) Perhaps more significantly, Francis Galton (1812-1911), the man who both coined the term "eugenics" and founded the eugenics movement, deeply admired Spencer and was influenced by Spencer's thinking on social evolution. Not so coincidentally, Galton was also the father of human population genetics, a statistical method designed to study patterns of inheritance as a way of explaining evolutionary developmental stages *within and between humans.*

Second, while Charles Darwin set the stage, it was Spencer, not Darwin, who developed the key concepts that would apply evolutionary theory to humans. It was Spencer, for example, who coined the phrase "the survival of the fittest."(5) Herbert Spencer was not focusing his ideas on the animal kingdom, but on social life, human behavior, and the internal *differences of evolution among humans.*

"As Humans Can Be Stratified in Evolutionary Development, So Can Cultures"

Spencer's influence upon a newly emerging field of anthropology, the "study of man," was also overwhelming.(6) Not only are humans to be arrayed along a continuum of evolutionary development, but so are the races and the cultures, societies, tribes, and nations in which they live. At an individual level, the idea of a "savage" or a "primitive" was at one end of that continuum and at the other was the "civilized person." So too, there was the notion of a primitive or savage society.

The fundamental basis of the continuum from savage to civilized, wrote Spencer, was the developmental stage of the brain. This was explained, in turn, by the way in which humans adapted to nature and, in particular, the seasons and the passage of time. The "primitive peoples" only had a sense of time relevant to such natural events as when birds migrate or when fall or winter or spring begins. The more advanced and more "civilized" could encompass decades, even centuries, into their thinking, planning, and "accumulation." As such, their brain capacity was vitally stimulated and, literally, enlarged. The longer the time sequence a human could encompass, said Spencer, the higher the level of intellectual development. At the bottom of the heap were the Australian Aborigines. Just above them were the Hottentots, who were judged one notch superior because they could use a combination of astrological and terrestrial phenomena to make adjustments to time sequences and changes (Spencer 1899). Moving on up, the next on Spencer's social evolutionary ladder were the nomads, just a rung below the settled primitives who lived in thatches and huts. Since they stored goods for future use, their conception of and relation to time was "more developed."

Anthropology, the new scientific study of human groups across all human societies, was born in this same period of evolutionary theory and was saturated by it. Just as humans can be stratified according to their social evolutionary developments, it was argued, so too can their cultures. It followed that, once selected individuals from "inferior cultures" came to live in "superior cultures," there would be a limit as to what their brains, of lower developmental capacity, could handle. Writing a century before this claim would be made again by Arthur Jensen (1969), Spencer noted in 1896 that black children in the United States could not keep up with whites because of the former's biological and genetically endowed limits, "their (blacks') intellects being apparently incapable of being cultured beyond a particular point" (Haller 1971, 124).

This reached its logical culmination in the work of James George Frazer (1854–1941), who produced *The Golden Bough*, a prodigious six-volume work that formally stratified cultures and societies along a continuum from simple to complex, from savage to civilized. Frazer posited a three-stage hierarchical theory, that human societies evolve from magic, to religion, and, finally, to science.(7) At the bottom of the hierarchy, of course, were "primitive cultures."

It is well known that Darwin's biological evolutionary theory was not accepted among the Christian clerics at the time.(8) Equally important for the birth of nineteenth-century scientific human genetics, the Church had fiercely contested not only the biological evolutionary theory of the ladder from lower creatures to humans, but the Church also had a strong vested interest in attacking the stage theory of social Darwinism. The idea that, over time, humans ascend to higher and higher forms of linguistic complexity, moral reasoning, and spiritual existence was counter to prevailing Christian theology. Four years before Darwin published the *Origin of Species*, Bishop Richard Whately published *On the Origin of Civilization*. Whately invoked a modern-day version of sociolinguistics to provide empirical evidence that humans had declined, not improved, over the millennia (Fraser 1990, 13). In the late eighteenth century, scholars had turned their attention to the origins of European languages. A body of work had developed indicating that there was probably an original common tongue that mothered Sanskrit, several Indo-European languages, and some Asiatic languages.

This theory resonated with the idea that a falling away from basic religious truths was the fate of humans (Fraser 1990). A fundamental tenet of Christian theology was that humans had declined, not ascended, over time.(9) It must be recalled that Christianity posited an early state of perfection and a "fall from grace." Thus, it was not an uncontested position to argue that, in the beginning, there was savagery and primitivism and terrible warfare and sacrifices. To place science at the apex of evolutionary developments of human cultures was at odds with a strong strain of thought among theologians. There was thus popular and clerical resistance to these ideas. Many groups had to be persuaded. Enter social Darwinism.

This was the social and political context in which James Frazer's *The Golden Bough* was published. One can now see some of the reasons for the author's fervid assertions of counter evidence that "primitive man" was an early, barbaric, savage being. Ludwig Wittgenstein understood this well. He cast suspicion on Frazer's motives for recounting stories of how terrible things are among "primitive peoples" in the following way:

> Frazer (tells) the story...in a tone which shows that something strange and terrible is happening here. And that is the answer to the question "why is this happening?": because it is terrible (Fraser 1990, xiii).

Wittgenstein was hardly alone in his attack on the tautological and self-serving presentation of data by Frazer. The eminent French social theorist Emile Durkheim also dissected the key architecture of Frazer's argument. Durkheim held that there was nothing "primitive" about totemic organization among the so-called primitives, but that instead this served complex and parallel social functions with what occurs in "advanced" societies (Durkheim 1957; Moret and Davy 1926).

The search for empirical evidence to document social evolution within homo sapiens is the subject of a full monograph superbly documented in Stephen Gould's *The Mismeasure of Man* (1981). Gould reveals the painstaking care with which nineteenth-century scientists sought to "prove" that the size of the skull could be arrayed along an evolutionary continuum, with white males at the apex. When they failed, they improvised, compromised, or "finessed" the data.

The Germination of Human Genetics in Social Evolutionary Soil: The Birth of Human Population Genetics and Human Mendelian Genetics

In evolutionary theory, the idea of the survival of the fittest captivated the intellectual and political interests of population geneticists, many of whom were trying to find an evolutionary tree *within* homo sapiens. Here we come to the intellectual birth of human population genetics, and the discipline's basic and recurring relationship to matters of social stratification in the substance of *what is being looked for*. The core enterprise of the early human geneticists was the search for evidence that there is genetic stratification, i.e., higher and lower forms of life, higher and lower forms of intelligence among population groupings among humans. The hand in glove with both physical anthropology and (pre-Boas) cultural anthropology was a near-perfect fit. *Within* a relatively ethnically homogeneous nation, such as England, this "search" took the form of seeking to explain class differences through genetics. Here, the father of the statistical correlation that we still use today, Karl Pearson, (10) was not just out on an expedition to see whatever he could find. Rather, Pearson was looking for something very specific: evidence that the least privileged, the poorest, and the low school performers were genetically destined.

Population geneticists, beginning with Galton and Pearson, were looking for signs of something called "human intelligence." They were on the explicit hunt for that which would help explain the *social evolution* of select subpopulations to the top of the social and economic order. (11) This quest for an evolutionary explanation of genius, gentility, and civility at the top was the corollary of the quest for an evolutionary explanation of trouble at the bottom. The target population of the early population geneticists, then, coincided with smaller socially configured subpopulations. (12)

A very different wing of genetics was that fathered by the Augustinian Monk Gregor Mendel in the 1860s. Rather than employing statistical analysis of traits and characteristics in a large population, this wing of genetics searched for evidence of the appearance of traits in offspring that followed "laws of inheritance" (e.g., Mendel's account of transmission through dominant and recessive genes). After laying dormant for many decades, Mendelian genetics was rediscovered in the early part of the twentieth century.

Population genetics was more popular in England, in large measure because of the overriding concern with social class as a stratifying practice. In the United States, however, where ethnic and racial differences would play a large role in any human taxonomy, Mendelian genetics held sway (Kevles 1985). From 1880 to about 1920, approximately a half-million immigrants per year entered the United States (Sibley 1953). This difference between the two nations has long been noted as a significant force explaining how and why social and political movements for change developed in varying ways. It is less well appreciated that the implications for the relative developments of the biological sciences and genetics may also have been influenced by the vastly different experiences of the two nations with ethnic immigration.

The significance of the notion of dominant and recessive genes was profound. It would mean that a single gene could account for some trait. Those who followed the Mendelian tradition could search through families to see if they could find evidence of these Mendelian laws of inheritance. While many genes do not follow such Mendelian principles, the kind of orientation to the research problem is important to understanding the direction the search for human genetic principles would take at this early juncture.

Galton and Pearson were actively hostile to Mendelian genetics and derided this conception of genetic transmission in humans as "atomistic" (Wright 1959). Since Galton and Pearson were after variations in human intellectual ability in large population aggregates, they found Mendel's laws on inheritance based upon dominant and recessive traits in family trees not only irrelevant but a diversion to be attacked (Dunn 1962, 2). In sharp contrast, the eminent American geneticist Charles Davenport (1866–1944) was a "super-Mendelian" advocate. In the early years, until even the First World War, there was considerable hostility and even open fighting between the population geneticists, mainly English, and the Mendelians, mainly American.[13] Nonetheless, there was a remarkable, even stunning convergence in much of what some of these researchers and their followers in the eugenics movement considered to be wrong at the bottom of the social order. The social and political interests of the human geneticists were intertwined with the questions that would in turn constitute the *fundamental building block of science*. Contemporary scientists are often drawn to make the separation between pure and applied science, and pure and applied genetics. But that is a distinction that is hard to sustain as one gets closer and closer to the decisions about what kinds of questions are to be investigated in human genetics.

Charles Davenport (1914), arguably the most influential American human geneticist of his day, was also a eugenicist. Davenport fused genetics and eugenics in ways that are, in retrospect, embarrassing. Most of the enthusiasts for human eugenics, then as now, were not formally trained practicing geneticists. Davenport, the esteemed biological scientist and an unreconstructed Mendelian, was unabashed in his embrace of eugenics. He went so far as to count up the number of male offspring from his Harvard graduating class (141), and when he contrasted this with the number of males in his class (278), he sounded the following alarm:

> Assuming that a class matures half as many sons as it graduates and that their descendants do the same for six generations, 1000 Harvard graduates in the 1880s will have sixteen male descendants of the 2080s. These sixteen sons will be ruled by the scores of thousands of descendants of 1000 of the Rumanians, Bulgarians, Greeks and hybrid Portuguese of the 1880s. Such figures must make one fear for the future (Davenport 1914, 11).

What Davenport feared was that these "lower forms of human life" on the evolutionary scale would someday rule the "higher forms" from the old Harvard stock. In its crudest formulation, this idea would take an ugly political and public policy turn—both the strong advocacy and the practice of forced sterilization of those at the bottom of the social order.

> The lowest stratum of society has, on the other hand, neither intelligence nor self-control enough to justify the State to leave its matings in their own hands. On the contrary, the defectives and the criminalistic are, so far as may be possible, to be segregated under the care of the State during the reproductive period or otherwise forcibly prevented from procreation (Davenport 1914, 10).

Ronald Fisher, generally credited appropriately as the founder of modern statistics, invented most of the statistics (between 1916 and 1932) now used in biological research, including the *analysis of variance.* Fisher was the author of a very influential book entitled *The Genetical Theory of Natural Selection* in which he proposed a theory of evolution. Published in 1930, the book sounded the familiar alarm (by that time) that since the lower classes were outbreeding the upper classes, the human species was in danger of deterioration (Schiff and Lewontin 1986, 10). Fisher's statistical genius created a *detente* if not a peaceful resolution between population and Mendelian genetics. With the analysis of variance, he developed a statistical strategy for assigning different weights to different causes, most particularly relevant, between "heredity" and "environment." But Fisher also used statistics to buttress and embellish Mendelian genetics.

> Simultaneously he was the inventor of the modern theory of quantitative genetics that shows how Mendel's laws can be used to generate the observed similarity between relatives in continuously varying traits like height, weight, and IQ scores (Schiff and Lewontin 1986, 10).

In order to appreciate better the continuity with the past, one must step back and place this development within the context of the great transformation in the social, political, and economic circumstances of the period.(14) At the turn of the century, hundreds of thousands of

Europeans were immigrating annually to the United States. During the three decades from 1885 to the First World War, more than 15 million Europeans came to the American shore as permanent émigrés (Sibley 1953, 382). Prior to 1885, European immigration had been primarily from England, Scandinavia, and Germany.

However, in the 30-year period prior to the First World War, the "new immigrants" were predominantly Italian, Russian, Polish, Slavic, and Jewish (the latter cutting across several national boundaries). The already-arrived groups (English, Scandinavian, and German-Americans) saw real threat in the new immigrants (Kamin 1974; Ludmerer 1972; Gusfield 1963; Haller 1963). Across many spheres of American life, the self-proclaimed "full-blooded" northern and western European-Americans pooled their resources and moved to collectively block further "alien" immigration. Ultimately, they would succeed. Congressional action in 1924 would slam the door almost completely shut on those from the southern, central, and eastern parts of Europe.

For example, yearly immigration from the Baltic states and Russia was 250,000 in both 1913 and 1914, but dropped to 21,000 in 1923, then dropped to 1,000 per year for the next 50 years (Lieberson 1980, 9). Similarly, Italian immigration dropped from 222,000 in 1921 to 56,000 in 1924, dropped even further in the next decade, and never again approached even the 1924 level.

The United States passed immigration laws in the 1920s that were unashamedly committed to racial and ethnic quotas, and nearly a half century was to elapse before they would be substantially repealed. The first restrictive legislation in 1921 set quotas at 3 percent for immigrants from any nation then resident in the United States. In congressional testimony to justify the new legislation to stop the flow of this "lower form of human life," the "scientific" IQ test became a powerful justification device. Jews (and Russians and Italians) had been revealed by the Binet test as genetically inferior, more prone biologically to "feeblemindedness."

> The mental testers pressed upon the Congress scientific IQ data to demonstrate that the "New Immigration" from southeastern Europe was genetically inferior. That contribution permanently transformed American society (Kamin 1974, 12).

In the next two years, Congress was besieged by eugenicists' testimony, arguing from IQ test data collected by the Army during universal conscription from the First World War. Just closing the borders of the nation was not enough. The eugenicists wanted to impose harsher quotas on the nations of southern and eastern Europe because the test scores were used to show that Italians, Slavs, Jews, and Poles came from inferior racial stock (Gould 1981, 232). They won the fight, and a new, more restrictive law was passed in 1924, resetting the quotas at 2 percent from each nation recorded in the 1890 census. Since northern Europeans and the British had predominated in 1890, this effectively shut off the "flood of immigration" from southern, south central, and eastern Europe.

This was part of the first great social and economic transformation of America from agrarian to industrial and urban society. The accompanying social troubles made for a receptive audience, among both scientists and laypersons. The problems of poverty, crime, mental retardation, and mental illness, it was asserted, could best be explained by reference to the qualities of the individuals who brought these problems with them, these "lower forms on the evolutionary tree" or from "lower forms of cultural life." Even the infant mortality rate was explained by reference to "qualities inherent" to those so victimized:

> The negro infant death rate is in every district higher than the white rate. Throughout the Austro-Hungarian and Russian districts, with very high density of population and great poverty, the infant mortality is exceptionally low. There can be no question that the low rate is due to the qualities inherent in the people themselves (*Eugenical News* 1916, 79).

As the United States and other industrialized nations now move into their second great transformation, from an industrial society to a service-dominated society, we are witnessing a similar set of social problems of high levels of endemic unemployment, high rates of homelessness, social dislocations, and the sense of less safe streets. As in the past, the pendulum must swing back and forth between explaining these developments by reference to the qualities and characteristics of individuals (and the societies or cultures from where they come) versus the social and economic forces that might also explain these "dislocations." In this swing of the pendulum, human genetics has always played an important role.

There are two fundamentally different approaches to the study of how knowledge develops in a society or culture.(15) In the first approach, the analyst looks at *which kinds of questions get raised,* and asks why. (The popular understanding of this is often illustrated with the observation that Eskimos differentiate between more than 40 kinds of snow,(16) while most who live in temperate zones distinguish between only three or four.) In the history of human genetics, one has seen how the saturation of social evolutionary thought prefigured many of the most important questions that would be raised for scientific inquiry.

A second approach focuses on the internal structure of knowledge, namely, the *rules of procedure for answering* these questions, the canons of evidence, strategies and techniques of investigation, the systems of categorizing, and the arraying of answers. The philosophy of science literature is dominated by the second concern (Gutting 1980; Kuhn 1962; Popper 1959; Kaufmann 1958). These are widely divergent approaches with sharply different conclusions and implications for one's ultimate position on either the bias or neutrality of knowledge formation. A concern for which questions get raised can be as fundamental as the concern for the rules of procedures for answering questions, with regard to the structure and outcome of knowledge development. An often-cited example is the extensive knowledge about the biochemical aspects of reproduction/birth control among women, but the paucity of knowledge about the biochemical aspects of reproduction/birth control among men. This has led some to the conclusion that a concern for the attributes of scientists might help explain what questions they pursue (the first approach cited above). Yet this is a different order of concern than a focus upon the forces, laws, and principles that accounts for why a bridge stands or falls (the second approach cited above). The latter has little to do with, for example, the race or gender of the engineer or physicist. In a similar vein, when it comes to medical training, there is something compelling in the argument that in performing a surgical operation, you have to know how and where to cut. However, if we back up a bit and raise a different order of question about the very foundation of medical research and training, we will see that knowledge formation is not so easily described.

The United States has one of the highest rates of infant mortality of any industrialized nation, even though it has a very high standard of living. The issue of what is appropriate medical research and training suddenly gets complicated, because while there may be only one or one best way of removing gallstones or performing an appendectomy, the *prior question* is whether medical students get trained to treat the gout or to remove gallstones, or whether the emphasis goes to primary prevention medicine. When the Western-trained medical faculties introduced the curriculum for medical students into Nigeria, the African students were being prepared to treat ailments of the middle and late years, while primary medicine and the relevant research to support it were badly neglected (Ashby 1966). In knowledge development for a society, priorities, emphasis, and choice mean that it is always a decision as to where to place resources, time, and energy.

Two different approaches to knowledge development can now be recast. One order of question is: How does one build a bridge, how is surgery performed, or how is intelligence measured? Even the most rigid positivist would grudgingly acknowledge the point that it is quite another matter (political) as to whether one builds a bridge here or there, performs surgery on the rich or the poor, or measures the intelligence of group A or group B. Many of the central questions that shaped the study of human genetics engaged the evolutionary paradigm. This is not to suggest that all or even most human geneticists were so engaged.(17) Indeed, the countering position is that human geneticists have also played a role in undermining false stereotypes about human qualities and their implications. Along with other scientists from hematology to neurophysiology, part of the legacy has been a corrective to popular misconceptions about human groupings. But the concern here is about raising a greater awareness of unexamined issues, some of which may be otherwise ignored because they are inadvertent or would remain unexplored precisely because in the "sole concern" with science, medicine, and health, the embedment of stratification issues are cast as irrelevant or political. This is especially a source of concern during periods of great social dislocation.

The Appropriation of Genetic Explanations

Of the many human attributes, characteristics, traits, or behaviors that "run in families" or "populations," why do some become prime candidates for a genetic analysis and treatment and are investigated with a program of research?

Those making the claims about the genetic component of an array of behaviors and conditions (crime, mental illness, alcoholism, gender relations, intelligence) come from a wide range of disciplines, tenuously united under a banner of an increased role for the explanatory power of genetics. For example, Edward Wilson is an entomologist who made his reputation studying insect societies (Wilson 1971). Yet he received the Pulitzer prize for publishing a book applying a genetic theory to social life of humans (Wilson 1978). Then, in *Genes, Mind, and Culture* (coauthored with Lumsden 1981), he went on to argue that culture itself is sprung largely from genetics. Arthur Jensen (1969), who vaulted to national fame with a claim on the relationship between genetics and intelligence, is an educational psychologist. Seymour Kety (1976), a psychiatrist, is one of the leading figures in the world espousing the *genetics* of schizophrenia. David Rowe (1986) and Sarnoff Mednick (1984), who argue the genetic basis of crime, and Eysenck (1975, 1971), who argues the genetic basis of psychopathology and intelligence, are all psychologists. Richard Herrnstein (1971) is a Harvard psychologist who has not only argued the genetics of intelligence but has even speculated that someday "the tendency to be unemployed may run in the genes." Herrnstein teamed with James Q. Wilson (1985, 103), a political scientist, to write a book that asks for a more sympathetic reading of the possible "biological roots of an individual predisposition to crime." And it is a sociologist, Robert Gordon (1987), who argues that race differences in delinquency are best explained by IQ differences between the races, not socioeconomic status.

Relatively few of these claims come from molecular genetics. Molecular geneticists, whether specialists with humans, animals, or plants, are typically wary of making claims about the genetics of these forms of human behavior. How can the relative modesty, scientific tentativeness, even quietude of these laboratory geneticists on these subjects be explained, while researchers in these other traditions of genetics tend to be the most passionate advocates for the biological or genetic component? It is the rare molecular geneticist who would stake his or her professional reputation on the genetics of "altruism," "intelligence," or "crime."

A review of authors of publications in *scientific journals in the field of human genetics* over the last decade would be a fairer assessment of the degree of disciplinary crossover. Toward this end, a bibliographic citation list(18) was generated and analyzed for author information, and a search of five major sources was conducted to obtain information about each author's professional background, including academic training and credentials.(19) As displayed in Table 1, a study of the scientific backgrounds of the authors of these articles provides one answer to the question of who is making the genetic claims.(20)

Table 1. Summary of Authors' Credentials

Area of Specialization	Number of Authors
Academic Degree (Ph.D.)	
Biochemistry	5
Biology	5
Chemistry	7
Genetics	6
Psychology	7
Zoology	10
Unspecified Ph.D.	17
Total Ph.D.	**57**
Medicine (M.D. and D.O.)	
General	49
Pediatrics	3
Psychiatry	18
Total M.D.s and D.O.s	**70**
Total Without Doctorate	**7**
TOTAL CREDENTIALS FOUND	**134**

It can be noted from the table that the majority of the authors come from fields outside of genetics. *Only about one-fourth could be regarded as credentialed in human genetics, cytogenetics, or a genetic field of any kind.* From one perspective, it should matter less that one is trained in a particular discipline and more that one is engaged in interesting and important research, using proper methods, controls, etc., whatever the training. After all, new developments in molecular biology have forced a realignment of traditional disciplinary boundaries. For example, biochemistry (itself a merger of disciplines) is more related to vanguard research in genetics today than 20 years ago. However, even taking such factors into account, well over two-thirds of the authors have research training that is far removed from the frontiers of molecular genetics, a very technical field. The great majority of the authors do hold a medical degree. A National Academy of Sciences study (1975, 161–179) revealed, as recently as the early 1970s, that medical schools rarely offered a single course in genetics, much less research training. While the situation has changed somewhat with more than half the medical schools now requiring one course in genetics, it can hardly be said that this constitutes preparation for research in one of the most technical fields in the natural sciences. Indeed, in the early 1980s, genetic counselors with only a master's degree were getting far more advanced training in human genetics than medical students.

The selection of genetic explanations for a range of troubling human behaviors constitutes an *appropriation* of the imprimatur of molecular genetics to the explanation of these behaviors, where the molecular genetic basis is not well developed or, more frequently, nonexistent.

Trouble at the Bottom: Continuity and Persistence

While many are aware of the gross human rights abuses *in the name of eugenics* (Kevles 1985) during the early part of the century, most of the current advocates, researchers, and celebrants of the putative link between genetic accounts and socially undesirable behavior (or characteristics or attributes) are either unaware of *the social context of that history* or are too quick to dismiss that history as something that happened among the unenlightened. Both formulations miss the special appeal of genetic explanations and eugenic solutions to the most privileged strata of society. Well into the middle part of this century, respected bankers, politicians, governors, university professors, and other respected professionals favored the sterilization of the "lower forms" of human life.

In 1912, the American Breeder's Association, an organization of farmers and university-based theoreticians, created a "Committee to Study and to Report on the Best Practical Means of Cutting off the Defective Germ Plasma in the American Population." It was a five-man committee, chaired by a prominent New York attorney, and having among its membership a prominent physician from the faculty at Johns Hopkins. At the 1913 meeting of the association, the report was delivered (Laughlin 1914, 12–13) and read in part:

> Biologists tell us that whether of wholly defective inheritance or because of an insurmountable tendency toward defect, which is innate, members of (select) classes must generally be considered as socially unfit and their

supply should if possible be eliminated from the human stock if we would maintain or raise the level of quality essential to the progress of the nation and our race.

California had one of the longest-running involuntary sterilization programs in the country. In 1927, a team of prominent and respected citizens was assembled to consult on the effectiveness of this program. They included Lewis Terman, the most prominent psychometrician in the country, David Starr Jordan (president of Stanford University), and S.J. Holmes, a distinguished geneticist from Berkeley. Covering the period from 1909 to 1927, this group generated a series of reports that produced "the first comprehensive 'proof' that sterilization was cost-effective and posed no significant medical harm to the institutionalized persons at whom it was aimed" (Reilly 1991, 80).

In the 1920s, two major legal developments would shape and be shaped by increasingly dominant views of "race betterment" through biological science and its applications. The first would be new immigration laws, strongly backed by the old American stock, to close off the immigration doors to those from southern and eastern Europe. It is well known and fully documented how geneticists and eugenicists provided vital testimony before the U.S. Congress in the early 1920s (see Ludmerer 1972; and Haller 1963). This resulted in the passage of two laws, which in effect reduced annual immigration from a surging high of approximately half a million to less than about 10,000 by the end of that decade.

This strategy was overwhelmingly popular among local politicians in several key states. For example, the Virginia legislature passed an involuntary sterilization bill in 1924 (30–0 in the Senate, 75–2 in the House), noting that "heredity plays an important part in the transmission of insanity, idiocy, imbecility, epilepsy and crime." That law gave superintendents of five state institutions the power to petition for permission to sterilize selected inmates.

On May 2, 1927, the Supreme Court upheld Virginia's involuntary sterilization law, opening up a floodgate of sterilizations in the United States. These sterilizations would become a model that would soon be adopted, expanded, and forever made infamous by Hitler's Third Reich (Reilly 1991). In July 1933, Germany enacted a eugenic sterilization law. The American eugenicists provided the intellectual and ideological underpinnings and were widely cited as the genetic authorities for this development. California was one of the leading states in the country in terms of its use of involuntary sterilization laws. From 1930 to 1944, over 11,000 Californians were sterilized under these laws. The Germans cited the California statute as a model (in 1936, Heidelberg University awarded honorary degrees to several key American eugenicists), but they took it much further. In the first year of the German program, 52,000 individuals were placed under final order to be sterilized, a development that was in turn hailed by American eugenicists. The best estimates indicate that from 1933 to 1945 the Nazis sterilized approximately 3,500,000 people (Reilly 1991).

Genetics, Crime, Violence, and Race

The major advances in human genetics in the last three decades have occurred mainly at the molecular level. The ability to detect a number of genetic disorders, even prenatal, has given impetus to the hope that therapeutic interventions will soon follow. The promise of these developments has helped to provide the rationale for the funding of the Human Genome Project, designed to map and sequence the full range of human genes. However, as indicated earlier, human genetics has several different traditions. Correlational studies have had a long history of attempting to link select *behaviors* to possible genetic explanations. The historical pattern has been associated with trying to find corrective programs for "trouble at the bottom." The connection being made today between genes and social outcomes is obviously less ominous than that which resulted in massive sterilization programs in the first part of the century. However, this should not blind us to the parallels to an earlier era.

In particular, one can point to the contemporary converging preoccupations and tangled webs that interlace crime, violence, race, and genetic explanations. So-called genetic studies of criminality have a heavy dependency on incarcerated populations. Thus, for example, one of the more controversial issues in the "genetics" of crime is whether males with the extra Y chromosome, or XYY males, are more likely to be found in prisons than are XY males. The first major study suggesting a genetic link came from Edinburgh, Scotland. While all 197 males in this account of prison hospital inmates were described as "dangerously violent" (Jacobs et al. 1965), 7 had the XYY karyotype. These seven males constituted about 3.5 percent of the total. But since the authors estimated that only about 1.3 percent of all males have the XYY chromosomal makeup, they posited that the extra Y significantly increased one's chances of being incarcerated. Ever since, a controversy has raged as to the meaning of these findings and the methodology that produced them. Notice the logic of such studies: They argue the genetic link to crime but rely primarily upon incarcerated populations. Incarceration rates are a function of incarceration decisions, a fact that social science research has long shown to be a function of social, economic, and political factors (Currie 1985; Skolnick 1966). While there is no consensus among scientists about the genetic predisposition of the XYY male to more violent, antisocial, and criminal behavior, Aubrey Milunsky (1992, 58) recently reported:

In a few score of reported cases, an XYY fetus has been unexpectedly diagnosed during prenatal genetic studies that were initiated because of advanced maternal age or other reasons. . . . In the United States, an informal survey by one of the leading researchers on XYY males, Dr. Arthur Robinson of Denver, showed that about 50 percent of parents elected to terminate such pregnancies.

In the last decade, America has been building more prisons and incarcerating more people than at any other moment in our history. Indeed, in the brief period from 1981 to 1991, the prison population in state and federal prisons increased from 330,000 to 804,000 inmates. That rate constitutes substantially more than a doubling in a single decade, *the greatest rise in a prison population in modern history* (Bureau of Justice Statistics 1992).

Converging on this development is the racial patterning of those arrested and serving time. A review of prison incarceration rates by race in the United States since the 1930s reveals a pattern that should give pause to anyone who would try to explain these developments by reference to the genetic makeup of the incarcerated. The gene pool among humans takes many centuries to change, but since 1933, the incarceration rates of African Americans in relation to whites has gone up in a striking manner. In 1933, blacks were incarcerated at a rate of approximately three times the rate of incarceration for whites. In 1950, the ratio had increased to approximately 4 to 1; in 1960, it was 5 to 1; in 1970, it was 6 to 1; and in 1989, it was 7 to 1 (Bureau of Prison Statistics 1991).

Even in the last decade there has been a dramatic change with respect to incarceration rates by race. This is true for many states and is most dramatically seen in Virginia. In 1983, approximately 63 percent of the new prison commitments for drugs were white, with the remaining 37 percent minority members. Just six years later, in 1989, the situation had reversed, with only 34 percent of the new drug commitments being whites, but 65 percent minority members.

This raises a fundamental concern for the methodology of studies that try to link crime to genetics. These studies take already incarcerated populations(21) and then "leap backwards" to some hypothesized genetic or chromosomal makeup, e.g., the XYY factor. To take a population in contact with select institutions of control (in prisons, correctional facilities, mental hospitals, mental health facilities) and then try to get at the "genetics" of the phenomenon by finding statistical significance where there is more of phenomenon A in the institution than outside the institution could be seen as neutral and value free. Yet when judges, lawyers, police, and mental health professionals make their judgments, they are making social judgments. Therefore, when "value-free" researchers find a much higher proportion of A in prisons than outside of prisons (in relation to the percent of A in the population), using the logic and methodology of the XYY studies, these value-free researchers seeking an account of the "genetics of crime" would conclude something very different about the biological or social "causes."

The Violence Initiative: Continuity with the Past Via the Irrepressible Link

In September 1991, the National Institute of Mental Health issued a program announcement with the title *Research on Perpetrators of Violence.* The announcement was explicit in its aim to further research on cost-efficient measures that might "prevent" violence.

> The purpose of this announcement is to encourage investigator-initiated research on the etiology, course, and correlates of aggressive and violent behaviors in children, adolescents, and adults. Through this announcement, the National Institute of Mental Health (NIMH) expects to support research that will improve the scientific base for more effective and cost-efficient approaches to clinical assessment, treatment, management and prevention.

In specifying the priority areas of research interest, the Violence and Traumatic Stress Research Branch specified that "studies may focus on risk factors and procedures that contribute to the occurrence and influence the course of violent behaviors (e.g., neurochemicals and neuroendocrines, parent-child rearing practices . . .)." The following is the summary language of one of the funded project's major aims:

> This research seeks to contribute to the understanding of the origin of serious and chronic aggressive and antisocial behaviors so that preventive interventions can be more effectively timed and targeted. . . . The project involves a longitudinal design in which 310 parent-infant male dyads from low SES backgrounds will be assessed when the child is 18, 24, and 42 months of age. . . .(22)

Yet another funded project describes its method of selection as follows:

> One-hundred and twenty Black third-grade boys will be recruited from 10 classrooms in the Durham, North Carolina school system. Dyad type will be assessed by pupil and teacher ratings of the extent to which pairs of boys in the classroom initiate aggression against one another.(23)

The focus on troubling behavior at the base of the social and economic order is, of course, quite old. There is the strong tendency for any successive cohort of scientists looking back on an earlier period, with the hindsight of a century, to find that previous work was deeply flawed. That will certainly be true as historians of science in the late twenty-first century look back at this period. One can profitably employ more humility about these vital issues of stratification, personal attributes, and behavior. That is certainly part of the reason why a small portion of the budget, 3 to 5 percent, has been set aside to address the ethical, legal, and social issues in the Human Genome Project.

A number of scholars have received seed money to plan and explore a study of human genetic diversity, "to get a snapshot of genetic diversity and how populations are related, and to probe human evolutionary theory—human origins, migrations, and expansions" (Roberts 1992, 1300). This is called the Human Genetic Diversity Project, and *human* evolutionary theory is very much a feature of the agenda. A team hopes to collect DNA samples on approximately 500 populations worldwide, taking blood samples from 25 persons in each group. Among the central questions to be asked is one that addresses "the origins of modern humans . . . the origins and nature of Bantu expansion, and when the first agriculturalists swept across much of Africa some 2000 years ago" (Roberts 1992, 1301).

It is understandable that there will be champions of a value-free neutral foray into these territories. Nonetheless, the persistence of human social stratification and the historical record of the idea of evolution internal to homo sapiens calls for careful monitoring, continuous scrutiny, and feedback on these early developments.

Notes

1. There are some missing links, and there are some leaps of faith, and, indeed, as unreconstructed creationists (and not a few hard-nosed empiricists) are happy to point out, some faith.

2. Spencer actually sold 300,000 copies of his books in the United States alone (Haller 1971, 128).

3. Objecting to an opinion from the majority, Holmes' dissent included the statement, "The Fourteenth Amendment does not enact Mr. Herbert Spencer's Social Statistics" (Seagle 1946, 417n).

4. This was from a letter written December 10, 1866, to Joseph Hooker (Darwin 1959). Four years later, Darwin wrote in another letter to E. Lankester that "I suspect that hereafter he (Spencer) will be looked at as by far the greater living philosopher in England; perhaps equal to any that have lived" (Darwin 1959 2:301).

5. Not aware of this history, current common sense and conventional wisdom unreflexively attribute this notion to Darwin, since it is now also vital to biological Darwinian theory of the evolutionary tree in the animal kingdom.

6. It is true that Spencer and Edward B. Tylor (1871), the author of a similar treatise about the evolution of cultures, each claimed priority and accused the other of plagiarism. Nonetheless, it is without challenge that Spencer was the most influential social thinker of his era.

7. Fraser did not posit a lock-step evolution. He acknowledged a zig-zag path to "progress" and liked the metaphor of waves sweeping up the shore line, constantly progressing even as there is receding at times.

8. Even into the late twentieth century there are still strong holdouts on evolutionary theory.

9. In the middle of the nineteenth century, the theory had prominent proponents who lectured at Oxford and other major universities in the West.

10. Karl Pearson was a late nineteenth-century English zoologist who later in his career became a statistician.

11. This was the era of measuring human head shapes. These kinds of scientific practices of this period have been well analyzed by Gould (1981).

12. Pearson had a special strategy. After getting school teachers to rank students for such traits as vivacity, introspection, popularity, and handwriting, he found correlations between siblings for these traits to range between 0.43 and 0.63. Since these correlations were about the same as those between siblings for physical traits, he assumed the traits were hereditary. Thus, Pearson "concluded that personality and intelligence too were predestined in the germ plasm before birth" (Haller 1963, 13).

13. In the years after World War I, a partial reconciliation and convergence would develop between population geneticists with their heavy reliance on quantitative measures of frequencies and the Mendelian geneticists. Today, for example, estimates of carriers for genes that might produce a genetic disorder come from such a merger.

14. This section is based upon a larger segment from my *Backdoor to Eugenics* (1990), where this argument is more extensively developed.

15. This position has been argued elsewhere and only the key issues are summarized here (see Duster and Garrett 1984, 1–37).

16. Current work in anthropology attacks this particular example as not factual, but it lives in the popular imagination as good an illustration of the point as we have. For aficionados of the problematics of the example, see Martin 1986.

17. Among many others, Kuhn (1962) and a host of students in the social studies of science have shown how "normal science" need not address a wide range of underlying assumptions, or even that bench scientists could well be engaged in work that directly countered those assumptions.

18. Generated by *Medlars II*. The list included 107 bibliographic citations in the area of genetics and the subareas of deviance and mental health.

19. *American Men and Women of Science*, two volumes (Physical Science and the Social and Behavioral Science) 13th ed., 1986; *ABMS Compendium of Certified Medical Specialists*, 1st ed., 1986–87; *Who's Who in America*; and *Who's Who in Science in Europe*. Locating information on the credentials and training of every author proved to be difficult. Despite problems in tracking areas of specialization for everyone, credentials for 134 of the 200 authors were found, constituting just over two-thirds of the entire population. In about one-third of the cases, only the degree granted could be determined, and not the area specialization. These cases were not included.

20. The selection of articles was intentionally biased away from anthropology, sociology, psychology, education, and political science journals, since this would have weighted the study more towards social scientists. Instead, the study was pointedly aimed to see who was making claims in the genetics journals. The articles were published in the *American Journals of Medical Genetics, Human Heredity,* and *Clinical Genetics.*

21. Or populations in contact with the criminal justice system.

22. Grant Number R29 MH46925.

23. Grant Number R01 MH38765.

References and Additional Readings

Ashby, E. 1966. *Universities: British, Indian, African.* Cambridge: Harvard University Press.

Bishop, J.E. and Waldholz, M. 1990. *Genome.* New York: Simon and Schuster.

Currie, E. 1985. *Confronting Crime: An American Challenge.* New York: Pantheon Books Inc.

Darwin, F., ed. 1959. *The Life and Letters of Charles Darwin.* 2 vols. New York: Basic Books.

Davenport, C. B. 1914. "The Eugenics Programme and Progress in its Achievement." *Eugenics: Twelve University Lectures.* New York: Dodd, Mead and Co.

Dunn, L.C. 1962. "Cross Currents in the History of Human Genetics." *American Journal of Human Genetics* 14:1–13.

Durkheim, E. 1957. *Elementary Forms of the Religious Life.* London: Allen & Unwin.

Duster, T. 1990. *Backdoor to Eugenics.* New York: Routledge.

Duster, T. and Garrett, K. 1984. *Cultural Perspectives on Biological Knowledge.* Norwood, NJ: Ablex.

Eugenical News. 1916. Vol. 1, No. 11:79.

Eysenck, H.J. 1979. *The Structure and Measurement of Intelligence.* Berlin: Springer.

Eysenck, H.J. 1975. *The Inequality of Man.* London: Temple Smith.

Eysenck, H.J. 1971. *The IQ Argument: Race, Intelligence, and Education.* London: The Library Press.

Fisher, R.A. 1930. *The Genetical Theory of Natural Selection.* Oxford, England: Clarendon Press.

Fraser, R. 1990. *The Making of the Golden Bough: The Origins and Growth of an Argument.* New York: St. Martin's Press.

Frazer, J.G. 1951. *The Golden Bough: A Study in Magic and Religion.* 6 vols. New York: Macmillan.

Gordon, R.A. 1987. "SES Versus IQ in the Race-IQ-Delinquency Model." *International Journal of Sociology and Social Policy* 7:30–96.

Gould, S.J. 1981. *The Mismeasure of Man.* New York: W.W. Norton.

Gusfield, J. 1963. *Symbolic Crusade.* Urbana: University of Illinois.

Gutting, G. 1980. *Paradigms and Revolutions.* Notre Dame, IN: Notre Dame Press.

Haller, J.S., Jr. 1971. *Outcasts From Evolution: Scientific Attitudes of Racial Inferiority, 1859–1900.* Urbana: University of Illinois Press.

Haller, M.H. 1963. *Eugenics: Hereditarian Attitudes in American Thought.* New Brunswick, NJ: Rutgers University Press.

Herrnstein, R.J. 1971. "IQ." *The Atlantic Monthly* (September) 63–64.

Hofstadter, R. 1955. *Social Darwinism in American Thought.* Boston: Beacon.

Jacobs, P., Brunton, A.M., Melville, M., Brittain, R., and McClemont, W. 1965. "Aggressive Behavior, Mental Subnormality, and the XYY Male." *Nature* 208:1351–1352.

Jensen, A.R. 1969. "How Much Can We Boost IQ and Scholastic Achievement?" *Harvard Educational Review* 39:1–123.

Kamin, L.J. 1974. *The Science and Politics of I.Q.* New York: The Humanities Press.

Kaufmann, F. 1958. *Methodology of the Social Sciences.* New York: The Humanities Press.

Kety, S.S. 1976. "Genetic Aspects of Schizophrenia." *Psychiatric Annals* 6:6–15.

Kevles, D.J. 1985. *In the Name of Eugenics: Genetics and the Uses of Human Heredity.* New York: Alfred A. Knopf.

Kevles, D.J. and Hood, L. 1992. *The Code of Codes: Scientific and Social Issues in the Human Genome Project.* Cambridge: Harvard University Press.

Kuhn, T.S. 1962. *The Structure of Scientific Revolutions.* Chicago: University of Chicago Press.

Laughlin, H.H. 1914. *The Scope of the Committee's Work.* Bulletin No. 10A. Cold Springs Harbor, NY: Eugenics Records Office 12–13.

Lieberson, S. 1980. *A Piece of the Pie.* Berkeley: University of California Press.

Ludmerer, K.M. 1972. *Genetics and American Society.* Baltimore and London: Johns Hopkins University Press.

Lumsden, C.J. and Wilson, E.O. 1981. *Genes, Mind, and Culture: The Coevolutionary Process.* Cambridge: Harvard University Press.

Martin, L. 1986. "Eskimo Words for Snow: A Case Study in the Genesis and Decay of an Anthropological Example." *American Anthropologist* (June) 418–423.

Mednick, S.A., Gabrelli, W.F., Jr., and Hutchins, B. 1984. "Genetic Influences in Criminal Convictions: Evidence From an Adoption Cohort." *Science* 224:891–893.

Milunsky, A. 1992. *Heredity and Your Family's Health.* Baltimore: Johns Hopkins University Press.

Moret, A., and Davy, G. 1926. *From Tribe to Empire: Social Organization Among Primitives and in the Ancient East.* New York: Alfred A. Knopf.

Popper, K. 1959. *The Logic of Scientific Discovery.* New York: Basic Books.

Proctor, R.N. 1991a. "Genomics and Eugenics: How Fair Is the Comparison?" In G.J. Annas and S. Elias, eds. *Gene Mapping: Using Law and Ethics as Guides,* 57–93. New York: Oxford University Press.

Proctor, R.N. 1991b. "Eugenics Among the Social Sciences: Hereditarian Thought in Germany and the United States." In J. Brown and D.K. van Keuren, eds. *The Estate of Social Knowledge,* 175–205. Baltimore: Johns Hopkins University Press.

Reilly, P. 1991. *The Surgical Solution: A History of Involuntary Sterilization in the United States.* Baltimore: Johns Hopkins University Press.

Roberts, L. 1992. "Anthropologists Cling (Gingerly) On Board." *Science* 258:1300–01.

Rowe, D.C. 1986. "Genetic and Environmental Components of Antisocial Behavior: A Study of 265 Twin Pairs." *Criminology* 24:513–532.

Schiff, M. and Lewontin, R. 1986. *Education and Class: The Irrelevance of IQ Genetic Studies.* New York: Oxford University Press.

Seagle, W. 1946. *The History of Law.* New York: Tudor Publishing Co.

Sibley, E. 1953. "Some Demographic Clues to Stratification." In S.M. Lipset and R. Bendix, eds. *Class Status and Power.* Glencoe, IL: The Free Press.

Skolnick, J. 1966. *Justice Without Trial: Law Enforcement in a Democratic Society.* New York: Wiley.

Spencer, H. 1899. *Principles of Sociology.* Vol. 2. New York: D. Appleton and Co.

Spencer, H. 1896. *The Study of Sociology.* New York: D. Appleton and Co.

Tylor, E.B. 1871. *Primitive Culture.* 2 vols. London: John Murray.

Wilson, E.O. 1978. *On Human Nature.* Cambridge: Harvard University Press.

Wilson, E.O. 1971. *Insect Societies.* Cambridge: Harvard University Press.

Wilson, J.Q. and Herrnstein, R.J. 1985. *Crime and Human Nature.* New York: Simon and Schuster.

Wright, S. 1959. "Physiological Genetics, Ecology of Populations and Natural Selection." *Perspectives in Biology and Medicine* 3:107–151.

7

Linking Genetics, Behavior, and Responsibility: Legal Implications

Norval Morris, J.D.

The organizers of this conference phrased four questions about the issues being addressed. How would evidence linking genetics to behavior or a predisposition to behavior affect our views of legal responsibility? How will the ability to predict and explain antisocial behavior affect the appropriateness of blame and punishment? What are the implications of increasing the ability to predict behavior in the absence of effective and appropriate responses to control it? How is the criminal justice system likely to use such tests and their findings?

Before plunging into these thickets, a general perspective on criminal responsibility may be appropriate. Following Karl Popper, the world is a "world of propensities" in which different individuals have base expectancy rates of capacities for, and likelihoods of, specific behaviors; but it is a world in which, despite these propensities, indeterminacy predominates. No matter how hard I tried, how well trained I had been from infancy, my DNA precludes my achieving Michael Jordan's altitudinal "hang time" in basketball. And, likewise, even those with DNA identical to that formidable athlete's have only a slim likelihood of achieving anything like his "hang time"—there are many, many other factors at work to achieve that lasting elevation. And so it is with crime, and with most everything else.

The pressures towards crime on some are very great indeed, their base expectancy rates of criminality very high, but successfully predicting individual behavior at short odds is most rare.

There is nothing original in that thought, but it is relevant to problems of crime and punishment. Society is not without experience in handling clear criminogenic adversities, obvious pressures towards crime.

It is likely that this experience will, since past is so often prologue, condition responses in practice to these four questions.

How Would Evidence Linking Genetics to Behavior or a Predisposition to Behavior Affect Views of Legal Responsibility?

Very little! We know now of links between personal and social conditions beyond the control of the criminal that predispose him (the criminal is almost always a "him") to crime and tend to treat them as relevant to the quantum of appropriate punishment and not to the determination of responsibility. Only in extreme cases is responsibility trumped by predisposition. On this basis, evidence linking genetics to behavior will only very exceptionally render the actor "not guilty," though it may reduce or increase the punishment for his criminal act.

Mental illness and mental retardation provide good illustrations. Unless psychosis or retardation reaches a stage at which the actor is believed not to know what he is doing, or not to know that his conduct is regarded as criminal, our criminal justice system holds him responsible for his crime. And even for those extreme and rare states of fundamental cognitive defects capable of denying criminal responsibility, compulsory controls are then imposed, not in the name of crime but justified by social protection and the provision of treatment.

Thus, mental illness and mental retardation, even when clearly part of the genesis of criminal behavior, are not given exculpatory effect, though they are generally taken into account in determining punishment. Mostly this works towards leniency of punishment; but if the defect be such as to give strong indication of a high likelihood of future serious criminal behavior, it may work to increase rather than to reduce the quantum of punishment. An example: The U.S. Supreme Court approved a jury verdict sentencing a man named Barefoot to execution, based on the testimony of two psychiatrists (one of whom had briefly interviewed him) that Barefoot was a sociopath and likely again to injure someone either at large or in prison. (See *Barefoot* v. *Estelle*, 463 U.S. 880 (1983).) Set aside the unreliability of the diagnosis and the unlikelihood of the prediction, assume they were respectively meaningful and accurate, and one can see how a strong predisposition to crime, beyond the actor's control, is treated in current jurisprudence.

A similar approach to responsibility and punishment for crime developed during the period when it was believed that males with XYY chromosomes were peculiarly prone to violence. Set aside the probable invalidity of this belief and consider what was made of it while it was regarded as reliable: There was no serious suggestion that such males should be any less responsible, as a matter of law, for violent criminal conduct; the only proposals were that such a proclivity should be taken into account as a matter of social protection in determining what punishments should be applied to such conduct. As a matter of practice, therefore, the proclivity would tend to increase rather than to decrease the punitive response, though as a moral matter it would be agreed that the criminal's moral responsibility may be less.

The same is true of social pressures to crime. Extreme poverty is not treated as a ground for exculpating the thief (unless, in some systems, it be starvation that faces the thief, and then only for very minor takings of food). Pressures towards crime are readily appreciated as being great on the neglected youth of an inadequate family in an inner-city slum; but no one suggests that such a youth should not be responsible in law for his conduct; human sympathy and understanding there may well be, but it will not lead to legal exculpation. And, in practice, the likelihood of the youth's further involvement in crime by virtue of those adversities for which he is in no way to blame will lead to an extension of our control over him by law rather than to any diminution of punishment.

What emerges is that only in extreme and very rare cases will proclivities to crime—physiological, psychological, or social in origin—have a reductive effect on legal responsibility; if anything, they will tend to increase rather than to decrease the severity of society's response to the criminal behavior. Unless the actor lacked total control of his actions, he will be held responsible for them and his proclivity to crime, whatever its origins, will tend to exacerbate rather than ameliorate his punishment.

This analysis is not an indictment of current punishment practices. Criminal law systems, defining minimum acceptable behaviors, necessarily attribute free will to the actor, except in extreme cases—and this is likely to continue while our social organization bears any resemblance to what now exists. Criminal law systems are intended to be socially protective even more than they can be subtly morally graduated.

A prime example of this priority of purpose is seen in the current wave of mandatory minimum sentences so popular with legislatures in this country. By its nature, a mandatory minimum sentence prefers social protection to ethically sound retributive assessment, saying as it does: Whatever the causes of this conduct, he must serve at least x years in prison.

If the genetic—behavior link can be confirmed as highly predictive of criminal behavior in some individuals, it is expected that a similar path will be followed here too and that the result will be an increase of punitive control over that person, the risk he presents being greater, although his moral fault may be less.

How Will the Ability to Predict and Explain Antisocial Behavior Affect the Appropriateness of Blame and Punishment?

"Blame" should be defined to encompass the process that St. Peter follows as he meets the suppliants before the Pearly Gates. With precisely calibrated moral calipers he measures how far the fallen have fallen and how far they have struggled to rise. He has an absolutely perceptive points system of moral assessment.

"Punishment," by contrast, is a product of imperfect human judgment; it is attributive and imprecise; it relates strongly to the harm that the alleged criminal has caused; and it fosters a search for a scapegoat for every major harm that occurs other than by Act of God.

Person A shoots at person B, the wind blows, he or she misses; that will attract a lesser punishment than if the wind had not blown and person A had killed person B. Yet the moral failure is identical. Person A drives too fast and is rewarded with a speeding ticket; person B drives identically fast but sheer chance leads to an accident in which someone is killed, and person B may well do time.

Blame is related most closely to moral fault; punishment is related most closely to harm encompassed. Generally speaking, legal systems require at least some degree of moral fault and some harm as a precondition to the imposition of a just punishment; but very low amounts of blame seem to suffice if the harm is great.

It seems unlikely that in the immediate future increased DNA knowledge and increased understanding of human behavior will lead to a situation where there will be understood to be such a low quantum of blame (so defined) that the actor will not be held responsible by the criminal law. Some current examples from the miserable jurisprudence of capital punishment may confirm this view. Recent cases in the U.S. Supreme Court have not disapproved of the execution of those found "guilty but mentally ill," of the severely retarded, and of children whose criminal acts were committed when they were aged 16 or 17. (For a discussion of these cases, see *Ford* v. *Wainwright*, 477 U.S. 399 [1986].)

What Are the Implications of Increasing the Ability to Predict Behavior in the Absence of Effective and Appropriate Responses to Control It?

Unfortunately, there are genuine dangers here. There is a very strong tendency in the dark annals of crime and punishment to overpredict dangerousness and to take excessive measures to prevent it.

The history of sexual psychopath statutes dealing with allegedly sexually dangerous persons is a fearful model. These statutes spread like a plague through the criminal law systems of the states in the second quarter of the twentieth century and still endure in a few states. Their broad pattern is this: One convicted of a sexual offense, diagnosed as a sexual psychopath (or is given some similar imprecise categorization such as "sexually dangerous person"), and said therefore to have a high propensity to commit a sexual offense in the future is not to be released until he is treated and cured of his sexually dangerous proclivity. These laws are based on a series of dramatic misunderstandings. First, the fact that minor sexual offenders ("peepers and flashers," in the jargon of the trade) do have a high likelihood of repetition of their conduct is used to classify all sexual offenders as peculiarly likely to recidivate—which is not the case. Further, the availability and effectiveness of treatment is assumed, and, even more astonishingly, our capacity to predict future criminal sexual behavior is taken for granted.

The stark realities of the relationship between true positive predictions of violence and the concomitant false positive predictions, clearly understood by the scientist, is a closed book to the legislator and is misunderstood in most of the case law. There is no group for whom there will not be at least two false positive predictions for every one true positive prediction. (On this, see the U.S. Supreme Court in *McCleskey* v. *Kemp*, 481 U.S. 279 [1987].) The consequential glaring injustice to the individuals held because others like them may commit crime is obvious; for every crime prevented there will, at our present level of knowledge, be at least three persons protractedly imprisoned, two of whom would not commit a crime of violence if released. And that grossly understates the reality of most similarly unjust detentions.

It is hard to think of a genetic condition that would not be productive of many more than two false positives for every true positive prediction of criminal violence. Likewise, though less dramatically, to the extent that the punishments imposed on criminals are designed to take account of their future "dangerousness," the moral problem of the false positive prediction obtrudes. This does not suggest that it is unjust to take account of "dangerousness" in setting punishments. It does suggest that such an accounting should never lead to the imposition of a punishment greater than is seen as deserved by the harm the criminal has already encompassed. Past harm should set the ceiling of punishment; under that ceiling it is not inappropriate to take into account the risk the criminal presents in the future to society. These matters are stated as dogmatisms; obviously they merit and have received extensive philosophic study and have attracted a huge literature, but the genuine dangers in this third question had to be confronted.

How Is the Criminal Justice System Likely to Use Such Tests and Their Findings?

DNA testing as an adjunct to the detection and conviction of criminals, and as an aid to establishing innocence, is a hugely promising technique that has not been adverted in this chapter, which, as directed, concentrates on issues of responsibility, punishment, and social protection.

Efforts to answer the first three questions have led to a quite brief response to this last interrogatory. The criminal justice system is likely to use DNA-established proclivities to crime, high base expectancy rates for certain inherited characteristics, much as it uses other knowledge about physical, psychological, and social pressures towards crime. "Not very well" may be the best answer; but there is more to it than that. There is understanding that criminogenic pressures for which the actor is not to blame lessen fault and "blame," but there is equally an understanding that those same pressures increase future risk of social "harm." Legal systems struggle already with a fair balance here; no easy equipoise has been reached. The same struggle will continue as the Genome Project increases our knowledge of human behavior and possibly our ability to influence it by just punishments and fair social controls.

8

The Genetics of Moral Agency

Ronald S. Cole-Turner, Ph.D.

When geneticists and ethicists meet, it is usually to discuss the *ethics of genetics.* What does ethics have to say about genetics, for example, about its research methods and applications? The object here is to reverse the order and to ask not about the ethics of genetics but about the *genetics of ethics.* What does contemporary genetics research have to say about the assumptions made in ethics?

When one speaks of ethics this way, inquiring into its assumptions, one is usually asking about metaethics or about moral theory. Thus, Richard Alexander (1987) entitles his book not "The Biology of Ethics" or "The Biology of Ethical Systems" but *The Biology of Moral Systems,* thereby indicating that the discussion is concerned with far more than the biological foundation of a particular code of ethics or of a set of ethical principles. Rather, Alexander addresses how biology can illume our capacity for engaging in ethics in the first place. Similarly, the concern here is about the genetics of morality since we are interested in what genetics might have to say about how we see ourselves, and others, as moral agents. In particular, how, in light of behavior genetics, can genes be said to cause behavior, and does this genetic causality circumscribe or preclude human freedom and moral responsibility?

Behavior genetics, a relatively new discipline, uses both population and molecular genetics to study the genetic basis for behavior. Part of the difficulty facing the field, of course, lies in identifying and quantifying behavior, particularly human behavior. Whether measuring intelligence or diagnosing a mental disorder, the precise measurement of behavior presents a serious challenge.

Once behavior is identified and quantified, however, behavior genetics seeks to answer two broad questions. First, does the behavior have a genetic basis? Pedigree and twin studies are used to pursue this question. Second, how does the genetic basis function? Some human genetic disorders that have an impact on behavior (e.g., Huntington's disease or Tourette syndrome) follow basic Mendelian patterns of inheritance. When this is the case, there is the possibility that the pathway between the gene and behavior might someday be sufficiently understood so that behavior can be altered. Other genetically based syndromes or traits of behavior (schizophrenia, intelligence) are the expression of many genes, which may never be precisely identified. If this is so, then it is unlikely that the multiple, interactive pathways among the many behavior-related genes, their products, and the environment will ever be understood.

Recent behavior genetics research indicates that differences in personality traits (extraversion and neuroticism), social attitudes, and even religiosity can be explained in part by genetics (Truett et al. 1992; Bouchard et al. 1990; Eaves et al. 1990, 1989; Plomin et al. 1990, 1988). This indicates that the wide central core of normal human behavior, and not just the rare deviations from that core, is explained in part by our genes. This further suggests that the human being as moral agent is genetically preconditioned. Later sections will ask what this recent research indicates about society's self-awareness as moral agents. Next, however, consider whether behavior genetics, with its finding that behavioral abilities are in part genetic and thus innately varied in the human population, poses a challenge to the idea of social equality.

Genetic and Social Equality

Francis Galton (1978) is often credited with taking the initial steps in the field of behavior genetics in the 1860s, and ever since, his work in this field has been surrounded by controversy. In part, the controversy arose because of eugenic applications, which ranged from limitations on immigration in order to preserve "racial hygiene" to genocide, and early behavior genetics was sometimes used to support these efforts (Kevles 1992). In addition, controversy has surrounded the suggestion that behavioral differences in abilities, especially cognitive, are in any way based upon innate or genetic differences, since this very suggestion was seen as legitimizing and thus reinforcing a stratified social order based on elitism, racism, or ethnic superiority, and so challenging the principle of equality upon which Western liberal democracy is established. Because rival scientific programs such as behavioral psychology explain human variation as the outcome of purely environmental differences, these rival approaches have been seen as more amenable than behavior genetics to the principle of equality of innate ability. It is altogether likely that behavioral or environmental approaches have been favored and continue to be favored over genetic approaches for ideological reasons (Loehlin 1983). A generation ago in the Soviet Union, the Lamarckian genetics of T.D. Lysenko enjoyed an ideological triumph over the Mendelian approach. According to Julian Huxley (1949, 182), there were two reasons: First, Lamarckism "holds out the promise of speedy control" over nature, especially agriculture. The second reason "is a dislike of Mendelism because it implies human inequality, and because it can be taken to imply human helplessness in the fact of genetic predestination" (184). The extent to which Western ideologies also favor environmentalism is a subject for further study.

Underlying more than a century of controversy are two questions. The first is whether a scientific measure of human competencies is *categorically different* from a social and ethical assessment of human worth. That is, are the two statements, "X scores higher than Y on most variables," and "X is a person of greater worth than Y," statements of logically distinct sorts? Is one a statement of fact and the other a statement of value? Is one a statement of science and the other a statement of conviction, whether ideological or religious? Or are they logically connected, such that the truth of the first statement has some bearing upon our assent to the second?

According to a leading textbook in behavior genetics, "We suggest that genetic and environmental effects on individual differences are scientific issues. Social equality, on the other hand, is a value—and a very important one. If examined closely, there need be no contradiction. . . . Equality of opportunity and equality before the law are independent of the scientific question of individual differences, regardless of their genetic or environmental etiology" (Plomin et al. 1990, 400).

Is it really the case that social equality is independent of measurable equality? Can we not measure what we value and value what we measure? Is not the labor of measuring an expression of the value we find in what we measure? The belief in the independence of the act of valuing from the act of measuring, articulated most strongly by Anglo-American analytic philosophers of a generation ago, is a distortion of the modern era that protects the myth of value-free science. The myth and its protection are under attack by historians and philosophers of science, for the most obvious of common sense reasons, namely, that one does value what one can measure.

Valuing and measuring must of course be distinguished from each other, but the distinction must not become so strong (as it was for the analytic philosophers) that these two mental acts are separated and thus pursued as if each were wholly irrelevant to the other. They are distinct, not just in research, but in a person's ordinary way of thinking whenever he or she alters the content of an act of valuing in light of data. But the fact that many are willing to alter the specific content of their values in light of data and that we regard it as intellectually healthy to do so indicates that though distinct, valuing and measuring are deeply implicated in each other. Indeed, one is motivated to measure because one values, as even the previously cited text recognizes: "Values undoubtedly do enter the scientific process from the beginning, when we decide what problems to study and when we interpret the findings and their implications" (Plomin et al. 1990, 398). But if that is so, then one does not have to wonder how to go about *adding value* to what has been measured, since one measured it having already recognized its value.

If this is the case, then it would be helpful to try to say in advance what values are found in the variables being measured through the methods of behavior genetics. David Hume recognized that people respond differently, not just to differing levels of ability, but variously to various competencies: "We may observe, that the natural abilities, no more than the other virtues, produce not, all of them, the same kind of approbation. Good sense and genius beget esteem: Wit and humour excite love" (Hume 1978 [1739-40], 608). What values are found in cognitive abilities or in social attitudes, and how does one respond to individuals known to exhibit one ability or another? In particular, if we want to maintain that social respect is accorded to every member of our species regardless of measurable competencies, then a convincing ethical argument toward this end needs to be developed. And we need especially to wrestle with the question of whether genetic and behavioral variation justifies substantial variation in the enjoyment of social benefits, like wealth. Do genetic variations make differing levels of income an inevitability, ameliorated but never removed by social or environmental policy? One needs to expect that the findings of behavior genetics will be used by some to support a fatalistic attitude toward social hierarchy and thus to challenge the effectiveness of social programs aimed at leveling environmental advantages. Advocates of behavior genetics can respond that, of all research programs, behavior genetics alone will tell us how much variance is environmentally based, and thus whether social programs to relieve extremes in variation have any hope of success. To make this argument, however, advocates of behavior genetics need to recognize that what they are measuring is valuable.

The second question is whether the finding of behavior genetics that variance in individual behavior is attributable in part to genetic variance can be extended to variance among racial or ethnic groups. For example, if individuals within groups vary in behavior because they vary in their genes, does genetic variation also explain variations in behavior among groups? Specifically, is the difference in intelligence test scores for racial groups within the population of the United States to be attributed to genetic differences?

It has been known for a long time that some genetic diseases, such as cystic fibrosis, sickle cell, and Tay-Sachs, are found most commonly in identifiable groups. In the popular mind, it is altogether possible that as behavior genetics makes a case for the genetic bases for intelligence and other traits, it will be assumed that the genetic bases for these traits are strongest in identifiable groups. Is this a fair inference? Based on current behavior genetics research, the answer is clearly no. One reason is that compared to the genetics of diseases like cystic fibrosis, the genetics of traits like intelligence is vastly, perhaps inaccessibly, more complex. But more important, the results of research to date, while strongly suggesting that genetic variance accounts for some observed *individual* variance *within* groups, do not extend to conclusions about group-to-group differences (cf. Plomin et al. 1988, 26). Any appeal to the findings of current behavior genetics research to support notions of group genetic differences in traits such as intelligence would be an improper inference. In order to understand whether genetics plays any role in accounting for variations among groups, one would have to know a great deal more, both about the complexity of the brain and of the relevant environmental factors that affect intelligence.

Nevertheless, both questions—namely, what relevance measurable differences have on social value, and whether genetic variation accounts for behavior differences among groups—are areas of traditional controversy that we should not expect to disappear anytime soon. These ideologically laden controversies will continue to affect the social context in which behavior genetics research is conducted. A long-term, global rise in ethnocentrism may be occurring. An extended, global period of growing disparities between rich and poor, both within and among nations, may also be happening. Regrettably, behavior genetics will no doubt be misused to encourage or defend both trends. One can guard against this misuse not by ignoring the problem or by presuming the independence of science from social values but by developing clear, countervailing ethical arguments in favor of the view that social respect be accorded to every member of our species.

Historical Perspectives on the Genetics of Moral Agency

Throughout the history of Western culture, virtually everyone has agreed that the environment structures the qualities of the person. Not surprisingly, great emphasis has been placed on nurture and education as techniques for altering the environment to achieve a desired structuring effect. Not everyone has agreed, however, that genes (or natural or innate factors, prior to our century) also structure these personal qualities. Dissenters have typically argued that if nature structures the person, the person is not free. This debate was first conducted by religious thinkers and more recently by philosophers such as Locke and Hume. In this section, this history will be briefly reviewed in order to understand more fully the historical context of behavior genetics and so to be able to incorporate its findings into a general perspective on human nature and moral responsibility.

At issue is whether there is an inherited human nature that structures the moral capabilities and predispositions of the moral agent. Almost from the beginning of Western or Latin-speaking Christianity, the answer of theologians has been yes. Tertullian (145–220) believed that because of the fall of Adam and Eve, the human race is tainted with a propensity toward sin, and this taint is transmitted through reproduction. Augustine (354–430) agreed, developing an elaborate understanding of human fallenness as a pervasive disordering of the whole human person, soul and will included. Augustine's rival in debate, the British monk Pelagius, was perhaps the first systematic environmentalist, since he argued that humans repeat the sin of Adam and Eve not because of nature but because of imitation. At the time of the Protestant Reformation, Protestant and Catholic statements generally agreed that an inheritable contagion afflicts the species, but it was the Protestant theologians who developed the motif with a pessimistic rigor. "We bear inborn defect from our mother's womb. . . . All of us, who have descended from impure seed, are born infected with the contagion of sin. . . . Adam so corrupted himself that infection spread from him to all his descendents" (Calvin 1960 [1536–1559], 247–249).

More than a century before Galton, John Wesley wrote that God created Adam directly but that the descendents of Adam and Eve are conceived and develop in utero through natural processes that God has established. "God does produce the foetus of man, as he does of trees; empowering the one and the other to propagate each after its kind; and a sinful man propagates after his kind, another sinful man" (Wesley 1978 [1756], 282). It is hard to imagine how Wesley could have found language more explicitly linking the structure of moral agency with genetic inheritance. This theme is repeated at the beginning of the twentieth century by the popular American theologian, Washington Gladden: "Disease, disorder, infirmity, both of body and mind, may be transmitted to offspring, and thus children may be born with predispositions to vice and wrong doing. . . . The children of drunkards do inherit from their parents a neurotic diathesis which predisposes them to intemperance" (quoted by Smith 1955, 176). In a widely used theology textbook of the same time, Augustus Strong appeals to the nascent field of behavior genetics for support: "The observed transmission not merely of physical, but of mental and spiritual, characteristics in families and races, and especially the uniformly evil moral tendencies and dispositions which all men possess from their birth, are proof that in soul, as well as in body, we derive our being from our human ancestry" (Strong 1909, 495). Strong refers specifically to Galton's *Hereditary Genius*, claiming that it "furnishes abundant proof of the transmission of mental and spiritual characteristics from father to son" (Strong 1909, 495).

Since the origin of this condition lies in an historic fall, Christian theologians after Darwin had to change either the concept of fallenness or its explanation. An earlier group (roughly 1860–1920) changed the explanation, either by appealing to Lamarckism to explain how an acquired trait (sin) could be transmitted by Adam and Eve; or, as in the case of F.R. Tennant, by recognizing that Lamarckism was not likely to prevail, and so arguing that our prehuman ancestry left the imprint of the beast deep within our nature. After 1920, other theologians such as Karl Barth or Reinhold Niebuhr reasserted both the great seriousness and the *human* basis for sin. Niebuhr revised the concept of fallenness from a disorder of nature to psychological and social disorders, which are environmentally enhanced but which originate in distinctively human anxiety. Shortly after scientists such as Darwin and Galton began to ask about the biological basis for the human moral life, religious leaders and other humanistic scholars backed away from the linkage between biology and morality. Most Western religious leaders today (including even the creationists who hold to the classic account of the fall as an historic episode in history) do not see the human person as genetically inheriting any morally significant predispositions. Most are thoroughgoing environmentalists, quite like professionals in secular social services. Ironically, earlier Christianity was dualistic but recognized that nature structures our moral agency, while recent Christianity is less dualistic but more environmentalist. Both these two conjunctions seem to be contradictory and thus apparently brought about by the force of other considerations.

More often than not, traditional Christianity focused only on human negative predispositions, labeling them collectively as sinful nature. Behavior genetics suggests that a full range of predispositions is inherited; sociobiology, too, suggests that evolution has produced both selfishness and altruism. Emerging philosophical or theological views of human nature, if revised in light of behavior genetics and sociobiology, will need to take into account the complexity, the nearly incoherent mix of altruism and selfishness, that characterizes the biological antecedents of human moral nature (cf. Cole-Turner 1993). Furthermore, Western religious and philosophical traditions have tended to assume that we all begin at the same starting point, morally speaking. Behavior genetics, of course, points out the variation in inherited predispositions. So here, too, Western traditions will need to be modified (Cole-Turner 1992).

On this question of the genetic structure of the moral agent, modern Western philosophy followed a course of development similar to that of religious thought. John Locke criticized Rene Descartes' view of innate ideas, arguing that each individual is born a blank slate to be written upon by experience. Thus, experience (or environment) alone provides the content of our ideas, although the mind is active in joining them together, as Kant argued later. Even today, Locke is sometimes seen as the major inspiration of empiricism in epistemology and of environmentalism in moral theory, even though he recognized innate variation in abilities (Loehlin 1983).

David Hume is particularly interesting because he attempted to introduce scientific modes of study into the field of ethics. In the original edition, his *Treatise of Human Nature* bears this subtitle: *Being an Attempt to Introduce the Experimental Method of Reasoning into Moral Subjects* (Hume 1978 [1739-40], xi). Based in part on the Western philosophical tradition of the virtues and vices as habits, Hume argued that, by nature, human moral agents possess innate sentiments of approval and disapproval. Ethics arises through cultural or artificial conventions, all of which derive their moral force not from reason but from innate moral sentiment. Good patterns of behavior into which one is trained are called "artificial virtues" by Hume; destructive or contemptible patterns are called vices. On this, Hume reflects a tradition that goes back to the Greek philosophers. But Hume adds that there are such things as innate patterns of behavior, which he calls natural virtues and vices (Hume 1978 [1739–40], 574–621; cf. Hudson 1986; Mackie 1980; Penelhum 1975; Kemp 1970). Typically, habits were seen as acquired; for example, MacIntyre (1984, 191) defines them as acquired, and indeed in the classic tradition it is the task of education to train the pupil in the acquisition of the virtues. Hume's distinction thus provides the most clear anticipation of a contemporary response of moral theory to behavior genetics.

While Kant is less empirical than Hume in his approach to moral theory, he also holds the view (contrary to some interpreters) that there is an innate human moral nature. While the category of will is central to his *Foundation of the Metaphysics of Morals*, Kant portrays the human agent as predisposed to all sorts of evil and selfishness, especially in *Religion within the Limits of Reason Alone*. Indeed, the autonomy of the will is the basis for rivalry and warfare that naturally characterizes the human situation (Rumsey 1990, 116).

Some aspects of the thought of Hume and Kant are open to incorporating behavior genetics into a broader framework of inquiry into the human moral agent. Other aspects are less open, and ever since their time it is these later aspects that have been the more heavily emphasized by Western philosophy. For example, Hume's natural virtues and vices have not been developed, but his view that moral sentiment, not reason, identifies the moral has been developed into moral subjectivism, according to which ethical statements are mere personal preferences. Kant's sober assessment of human nature, troublesome to Enlightenment optimism, has been ignored in favor of the autonomous will, so unfettered as to have no constraints of nature, even to the point of existentialists such as Sartre holding that by sheer will, human nature is created. So Western moral philosophy in this century has typically portrayed the human moral subject as pure will, natureless, proposing its own essence and entitled to express whatever opinion it feels it likes.

In Hume's view, human moral agents have virtues and vices, or helpful and hurtful patterns of behavior, that are both innate and acquired; and, in either case, virtues and vices predispose one to certain types of action without necessitating any specific action. Can these ideas be brought into conversation with current behavior genetics research? When behavior genetics finds that variation in social attitudes is explained by variation in genes and environment, is it finding the empirical surface of innate and acquired virtues and vices? How, in other words, does one translate a scientific research program like behavior genetics into the language of philosophy and moral theory?

At the genetic level, according to behavioral genetics, there seems to be something like a predisposition to a disease or to resistance to a disease, a kind of presymptomatic diagnosis, but one that inclines us toward broad patterns of behavior or attitude. Genes, always interacting with complex environmental factors, give rise to predispositions that structure the moral agent, defining its usual patterns of behavior but in such a way that preserves the consciousness of choice and responsibility. This moral structuring, to which genes and environment contribute, defines what might be called the *moral phenotype* of the human moral agent. Traditional Western ethics often employed the category of *character* to identify the persisting moral patterns that define a person. Now in light of behavior genetics, character can be reinterpreted as moral phenotype. Behavior genetics seems to be well on its way in providing prima facie evidence for presence of the moral phenotype, which, like biological phenotype, is the structure that is expressed by genes interacting with the environment. No longer can moral theories ignore the biological and specifically genetic dimension of humanity by considering only a nonnatural, nongenetic will, structured only by its environment, if at all.

Genetics and Determinism

But if so, are we then faced with "genetic determinism"? That is to say, if it is true that the human agent is morally predisposed in part by genes, are we confronted with a genetic determinism that precludes freedom and relieves us of moral responsibility? For many, any notion of genetic determinism is to be rejected as incompatible with the assumption of moral responsibility upon which civilization is built. "The theory of an inherited second nature is . . . clearly destructive of the idea of responsibility" (Niebuhr 1942, 262). Does behavior genetics pose such a threat? In order to address this question, first, the sense in which it is being said that genes cause behavior needs to be carefully considered.

Behavior genetics indicates that measurable variations in behavior among human beings correlate with genetic variations. Does such correlation imply causality? More precisely, does behavior genetics show that differences in genes *cause differences* in behavior? One recent textbook in behavior genetics uses the term "cause" without hesitation: "Our book tries to analyze the genetic and environmental causes of the [behavioral] differences" (Eaves et al. 1989, vii). Another, only slightly more cautiously, asserts that correlation implies cause: "Correlations can be used to imply causation, despite the revered rule to the contrary. . . . We do not hesitate to impute causation to these correlations" (Plomin et al. 1988, 29).

Here, "causation" seems to mean more than Hume's sense of a mental association of the two observed factors, namely, genes and behavior. A stronger sense of "cause" is being claimed, in which genes (with environment) have the power to bring about the behavior. While the precise causal pathways (which involve not only the environmental factors but also the staggering complexity of the human brain) are not yet well understood, and may never be fully understood, biochemical pathways nonetheless connect genes to behavior in such a way that the genes in part produce the behavior. Behavior genetics is thus *deterministic in this sense*. Genes interacting with the environment determine patterns of behavior and social attitude. This does not assume or entail a metaphysical determinism, according to which all events are necessitated by antecedent events. Deterministic causality in behavior genetics is limited to the way in which genes, interacting with other complex processes, bring about and thus limit or determine the possibilities of the phenotype.

Nevertheless, behavior geneticists resist the term "genetic determinism," preferring softer terms. "The term 'genetic influence' does not imply that the environment is unnecessary for development, nor does it imply genetic determinism" (Plomin et al. 1988, 27). Why is it not deterministic? Because "no specific genetic mechanism or gene-behavior pathways are implied" (27). Certainly, "gene-behavior pathways" are not yet understood. But are they not implied and, indeed, the focus of research? It seems quite likely that the pathway between genes and behavior will be increasingly understood, so that human behavior will increasingly be explained on the basis of the understanding of genes and of all the factors with which they interact. Will this amount to "genetic determinism"? Not in a strict sense, since genes alone do not determine behavior. Instead, there is a "genetic-plus-environmental determinism" in which genes and environmental factors interact to determine the phenotype, including what can be called the moral phenotype.

Determinism and Responsibility

Does this determinism preclude human moral responsibility? The discussion of this question moves beyond the scope of behavior genetics, although research at this level greatly illumes the discussion and rules out some possibilities. Ruled out, for example, is the view that human beings are free to act in a way that is wholly unaffected by innate or genetic factors. But if one now sees his or her behavior as determined by the complex interaction of genes plus environment, is moral responsibility negated? To explore this question, other fields of inquiry must finally be brought to bear. These include the full range of the human sciences, together with philosophical consideration of the meaning of determinism.

A helpful philosophical distinction is between freedom as indeterminacy and freedom as the power of self-determination. If one thinks of freedom as indeterminacy and regards as free only those actions that have no cause, then of course behavior genetics (with other fields) challenges the ideas of freedom and responsibility, since behavior genetics sees actions as causally determined by, among other things, genes. The widespread tendency to think of freedom as indeterminacy may account for the widespread apprehensiveness about "genetic determinism" as the negation of human freedom.

If, on the other hand, freedom is thought of as self-determination, then it may be possible to reconcile freedom with the belief that genes and the environment determine behavior. This will depend on whether modern-day man can make sense of the notion of self-determination, as earlier philosophers such as Thomas Reid attempted to do. In the earlier version of the argument, it was granted that all events have causes that determine them, but the human self or person is the self-moved cause that determines human moral action. Such action is free not because it is uncaused but because it is caused by the self as moral agent. In light of behavior genetics and other fields such as brain research, is it possible to think of the person as a self-moved cause? Certainly not in the sense that the person-as-cause operates independently of other causes, contradicting them or limited to gaps of indeterminateness in their comprehensiveness. Instead, the person or moral agent should be seen as the complexity of the whole human organism that acts always within the determinations of the genetic and environmental constraints, but in a way that achieves not merely the consciousness of choice but also allows the organism as a whole to choose at any moment a concrete option from within the limits defined by genetic and environmental determinants. While behavior genetics and related fields certainly do not require that we see ourselves as agents of this sort, it could be argued that this view is compatible with findings from these fields of research.

For some, the very phrase "genetic determinism" conjures an aura of inevitability, inasmuch as genes are fixed at the beginning. They link humans with their ancestry all the way to the prehuman. Thus seen, genes appear to some to lock us into a vast web of biological determinism that deprives us of what distinguishes us from the rest of nature and so removes what we once thought was essentially human. By contrast, it has been argued that far from posing an ominous threat to humanity, behavior genetics and related fields of research offer to illume more precisely the moral nature of the human situation.

References

Alexander, R.D. 1987. *The Biology of Moral Systems*. Hawthorne, NY: Aldine de Gruyter.

Augustine. 1984. *Concerning the City of God Against the Pagans*. Translated by H. Bettenson. New York: Penguin Books.

Barth, K. 1956. *Church Dogmatics*. Vol. IV, 1. *The Doctrine of Reconciliation*. Translated by G.W. Bromiley. Edinburgh: T. & T. Clark.

Blum, K., Noble, E.P., Sheridan, P.J., Montgomery, A., Ritchie, T., Jagadeeswaran, P., Nogami, H., Briggs, A.H., and Cohn, J.B. 1990. "Allelic Association of the Human Dopamine D_2 Receptor Gene in Alcoholism." *Journal of the American Medical Association* 263:2055–2060.

Bolos, A.M., Dean, M., Lucas-Derse, S., Ramsburg, M., Brown, G.L., and Goldman, D. 1990. "Population Pedigree Studies Reveal a Lack of Association Between the Dopamine D_2 Receptor Gene and Alcoholism." *Journal of the American Medical Association* 264:3156–3160.

Bouchard, T.J., Jr., Lykken, D.T., McGue, M., Segal, N.L., and Tellegen, A. 1990. "Sources of Human Psychological Differences: The Minnesota Study of Twins Reared Apart." *Science* 250:223–228.

Calvin, J. 1960. *The Library of Christian Classics*. Institutes of the Christian Religion, Vol. 20. Translated by F.L. Battles. Philadelphia: Westminster Press.

Cole-Turner, R.S. 1993. *The New Genesis: Theology and the Genetic Revolution*. Louisville: Westminster/John Knox Press.

Cole-Turner, R.S. 1992. "Religion and the Human Genome." *Journal of Religion and Health* 31:161–173.

Cole-Turner, R.S. 1989. "Genetic Engineering: Our Role in Creation." In J. Mangum, ed., *The New Faith-Science Debate*, 68–75. Minneapolis: Fortress Press.

Darwin, C. 1968. *On the Origin of Species by Means of Natural Selection*. Baltimore: Penguin Books.

Eaves, L.J., Eysenck, H.J., and Martin, N.G. 1989. *Genes, Culture and Personality: An Empirical Approach*. London: Academic Press.

Eaves, L.J., Martin, N.G., and Heath, A.C. 1990. "Religious Affiliation in Twins and Their Parents: Testing a Model of Cultural Inheritance." *Behavior Genetics* 20:1–22.

Fairbairn, A.M. 1902. *The Philosophy of the Christian Religion.* New York: Hodder & Stoughton.

Flew, A. 1989."'Morality and Determinism': Two Comments." *Philosophy* 64:98–103.

Galton, F. 1978. *Hereditary Genius: An Inquiry into its Laws and Consequences.* New York: St. Martin's Press.

Hahn, M.E., Hewitt, J.K., Henderson, N.D., and Benno, R. 1990. *Developmental Behavior Genetics: Neural, Biometrical, and Evolutionary Approaches.* New York: Oxford University Press.

Hudson, S.D. 1986. *Human Character and Morality: Reflections from the History of Ideas.* Boston: Routledge & Kegan Paul.

Hume, D. 1978. *A Treatise of Human Nature.* 2d ed. Oxford: Clarendon Press.

Huxley, J. 1969. *Heredity East and West: Lysenko and World Science.* New York: Kraus Reprint.

Kant, I. 1960. *Religion Within the Limits of Reason Alone.* Translated by T.M. Greene and H.H. Hudson. New York: Harper & Row.

Kemp, J. 1970.*Ethical Naturalism: Hobbes and Hume.* London: Macmillan.

Kevles, D.J. 1992. "Out of Eugenics: The Historical Politics of the Human Genome." In D.J. Kevles and L. Hood, eds., *The Code of Codes: Scientific and Social Issues in the Human Genome Project,* 3–36. Cambridge: Harvard University Press.

Loehlin, J.C. 1983."John Locke and Behavior Genetics." *Behavior Genetics* 13:117–121.

MacIntyre, A. 1984.*After Virtue: A Study in Moral Theory.* 2d ed. Notre Dame, IN: University of Notre Dame Press.

Mackie, J.L. 1980. *Hume's Moral Theory.* London: Routledge & Kegan Paul.

Midgley, M. 1981. *Heart and Mind: The Varieties of Moral Experience.* Brighton, England: Harvester Press.

Niebuhr, R. 1942. "Human Nature." In *The Nature and Destiny of Man.* The Gifford Lectures, Vol. 1. New York: Charles Scribner's Sons.

Penelhum, T. 1975. *Hume.* New York: St. Martin's Press.

Plomin, R. 1990. "The Role of Inheritance in Behavior." *Science* 248:183–188.

Plomin, R., DeFries, J.C., and David, W.F. 1988. *Nature and Nurture During Infancy and Early Childhood.* Cambridge: Cambridge University Press.

Plomin, R., DeFries, J.C., and McClearn, G.E. 1990. *Behavioral Genetics: A Primer.* 2d ed. New York: W.H. Freeman.

Rumsey, J.P. 1990. "Agency, Human Nature and Character in Kantian Theory." *Journal of Value Inquiry* 24:109–121.

Smith, H.S. 1955. *Changing Conceptions of Original Sin: A Study in American Theology Since 1750.* New York: Charles Scribner's Sons.

Strong, A.H. 1907. *Systematic Theology*, Vol. 2. *The Doctrine of Man.* Philadelphia: Griffith & Rowland Press.

Tennant, F.R. 1908. *The Origin and Propagation of Sin.* Cambridge University Press.

Truett, K.R., Eaves, L.J., Meyer, J.M., Heath, A.C., and Martin, N.G. 1992. "Religion and Education as Mediators of Attitudes: A Multivariate Analysis." *Behavior Genetics* 22:43–62.

Wassermann, G.D. 1988. "Morality and Determinism." *Philosophy* 63:211–230.

Wesley, J. 1978. "The Doctrine of Original Sin, According to Scripture, Reason, and Experience." In *The Works of John Wesley IX.* Grand Rapids, MI: Baker Book House.

Zahn-Waxler, C.E., Cummings, M., and Iannotti, R., eds. 1986. *Altruism and Aggression: Biological and Social Origins.* Cambridge: Cambridge University Press.

Zuckerman, M. 1990. "Some Dubious Premises in Research and Theory of Racial Differences: Scientific, Social, and Ethical Issues." *American Psychologist* 45:1297–1303.

PART IV

Genetic Testing and Determination of Property Rights

INTRODUCTION

The Scope and Value of Patent Protection

Gilbert S. Omenn, M.D., Ph.D.

Benjamin Franklin introduced the concept of protection of intellectual property—inventions and discoveries—and Article 8 of the U.S. Constitution provides for patents to promote the progress of science and the useful arts. Patents have proved valuable in the emerging biotechnology industry as well as in the pharmaceutical industry to assure companies of a defined period in which to gain financial return on the huge up-front investment in drug development and clinical trials required to demonstrate efficacy and safety for the select few agents that prove clinically useful. In other industries, trademarks, copyrights, and trade secrets have functioned in place of patents and licenses.

Kate Murashige provides an excellent overview of the nature of the intellectual property protection offered by the patent system. She outlines the unusual features in its application to living organisms (the Chakrabarty oil-eating bacterium, the Harvard mouse) and gene sequences (the Venter/NIH filings for thousands of "expressed sequence tags" from a library of human cDNAs). Applicants and the U.S. Patent and Trademark Office are continuing to define the scope of enforceable patent protection—broad enough to be effective, but not so broad as to preclude subsequent innovation. Most importantly, Murashige and Thomas White explain that a patent is only an opportunity to assert one's priority, with sometimes daunting costs to do so. The biotechnology industry has already had more than its share of costly patent battles as patents have been issued on a case-by-case basis that leaves the resolution of priority to "interference proceedings," legal battles that follow the issuance of the patents. Now university researchers, as well as industry research and development units, are worried that patent-holders will seek to enforce claims of infringement on anyone using a patented material or process without paying fees to do so. Discussions about potential exemptions from infringement for "research purposes" are an important element of all the chapters in this section. To provoke discussion, the authors raise a question about whether patents that restrict others from using a valuable product or process or living organism should even be allowed.

Examination of the fundamental aims and boundaries of patent rights is being accelerated currently by efforts at harmonization of the approaches in the United States with those in Europe, Canada, and Japan. The differences are very large, beginning with the criterion for defining who has priority for an invention. In the United States, it is the first to discover or invent, which is complicated to prove in many cases and requires documentation in laboratory notes and great care about what is stated at meetings or published in any form. In Europe, priority goes to the first to file a patent application. Even then there must be a judgment about what are independent claims.

Thomas White focuses on the furor caused by the NIH decision to seek patents on the thousands of partial gene sequences from Venter's cDNA method. He provides a very useful summary of biotechnology advances that have been patented and others that have not been patented. He concludes that many of these advances have been of great benefit to research, medicine, society, and companies, regardless of the patent situation. Also, he cites examples in which basic and applied research were not inhibited by patenting of processes. He analyzes the likely impact of certain proposed changes, such as requiring that function be known, or patenting uses of genes, or requiring that sequences be deposited in publicly accessible gene banks.

Joan Overhauser presents the viewpoint of a university scientist apparently not involved with any companies. She notes the burden already growing from "material transfer agreements" some scientists are requiring before sharing their biological samples. She also makes clear that modern collaborative research, especially on clinical problems, requires many other key contributions besides those of the individual or firm that invents or discovers a particular product or process for diagnosis, treatment, or prevention of a clinical disorder. Finally, she raises the specter of skyrocketing medical expenditures and suggests that DNA patenting will add to that problem.

Ted Peters focuses on the NIH/Venter cDNA patent applications in responding to the Murashige chapter. His criterion is globally framed: "Insofar as patent protection encourages the worldwide flow of information that enhances research everywhere—especially research aimed at improving human health and well-being—it is desirable. . . ." Then he reinforces the common ethics analysis that somatic gene therapy may be judged like any other medical intervention, while germline interventions raise justifiable fears of mischief or of mistakes and, at least, of hubris.

These chapters should help the reader understand the background of patenting in the biopharmaceutical field. As a university scientist with involvements in the biotechnology industry, it is important to point out that patenting has been considered a lifeline for emerging companies whose up-front investment and brilliant scientific and clinical findings might otherwise be pirated by others. At the same time, confusion about what can be patented, the high cost of defending one's patents, the conflicting international criteria for patents, and the sense of affront many citizens may feel about patenting genes or organisms (let alone humans!) as they occur in nature should stimulate fresh thinking about the role and means of protection of intellectual property in science generally and in genetics in particular.

9

Intellectual Property and Genetic Testing

Kate H. Murashige, J.D., Ph.D.

It is probably no longer surprising that the elements and tools involved in genetic testing, and the overall methods used in some genetic tests per se, can be the subject of intellectual property protection. It may also not be surprising that methods for genetic manipulation and the end products thereof (which may well constitute the justification for genetic testing as well as having utility in and of themselves) are the subjects of intellectual property protection. To the extent that genetic testing and the genetic engineering "repairs" or other modifications occasioned by the results of the testing can be thought to be components of the general economic system that uses monetary incentives to encourage research efforts, such intellectual property protection is appropriate. The correctness of including such endeavors within the general market-driven framework of a capital-based economic system, as opposed to replacing these mechanisms with some alternative, is clearly open to debate.

Specifically, recognition is rapidly growing that health-related services have become a "medical-industrial complex" and that the operation of this market-based system has resulted in escalating costs and an unjust distribution of services. Genetic testing and manipulation may be more subject to scrutiny than many other more commonplace health services. It may be, therefore, that a less profit-oriented and money-driven mechanism, more akin to universal health insurance or socialized medicine, will emerge. To the extent this occurs, intellectual property protection as a vehicle for acquisition of liquid or other nonintellectual assets becomes less important.

This chapter contains four major subsections in advance of a general conclusory section summarizing the questions left open by consideration of the issues raised in the text. These subsections address

1. the nature of intellectual property

2. the manner in which protection for elements of genetic testing and manipulation has been sought

3. the reasons this protection raises questions not present in other areas of intellectual property

4. policy issues that have been raised in connection with this subject matter

The Nature of Intellectual Property

The concept of "property" in general is so much a part of Western society that to attempt to define it seems as useless as to attempt to define "life." It might be useful at the outset to remember that property cannot exist without a system of ascribing rights to certain individuals or groups as "owners" with respect to certain subject matters. The nature of the subject matter and the rights of the owner varies greatly. The subject matter may be land or tangible property where, depending on its precise nature, the owner may have a plethora of rights limited only by considerations with respect to the values of society as a whole. For example, an individual may own a dog but, at least in a well-ordered society, may not mistreat it; a person or a corporation may own land but may not use it for purposes that contravene zoning laws or public safety. Ownership of property, therefore, confers a set of rights with respect to owned subject matter that are never absolute.

The rights conferred on the owners of intellectual property are perhaps more explicitly defined and less comprehensive than the rights enjoyed by owners of other property. Intellectual property may differ from tangible personal property or real property in that the system designed to define the rights of the owner also defines the subject matter of the ownership. One does not need a statute to define the *subject matter* owned when that subject matter is a house, a car, or a box of stationery. However, with respect to intellectual property, the subject matter that can be owned, as well as the nature of the ownership, is defined by the legal system. The patent system, for example, does not provide for "ownership" of an algorithm or a natural law; and a potential "owner" must define the nature of, for example, a composition of matter that is to be claimed.

The four recognized types of intellectual property protection so far devised by various societies and jurisdictions include trademark, trade secret, copyright, and patent. The first three are of little relevance to genetic testing or genetic techniques, so there is little point in discussing them much further. There has been some suggestion that copyright protection could be appropriate for the protection of gene sequences;

however, this concept seems to have fallen into the shadows over the last 10 years or so. It may be worth some further consideration in view of the massive efforts exerted in connection with the Human Genome Project. It would be a major intellectual challenge to consider how the copyright system might effectively protect gene sequences. Copyright confers protection of an author's expression, not of an idea per se; furthermore, copyright does not protect against independent discovery or creation. From time to time, certain aspects of genetic testing and engineering have been considered as subject matter for trade secret protection, but this too seems not to have become a major avenue for participants in the field. Right now, patents seem to be king. Therefore, it may be helpful to be reminded of the elements of this system.

In the United States, the statutes that define the subject matter and rights of owners of intellectual property protected by patents are contained in Title 35 of the U.S. Code. The rules governing the granting of patent rights to applicants are in Volume 37 of the Code of Federal Regulations. The nature of the subject matter and rights conferred in the United States are similar, but not identical, to those provided for by statute in other jurisdictions. Attempts to harmonize the patent laws of at least the United States, Europe, Japan, Canada, and other industrialized nations have been the subject of increased activity in several contexts—trilateral negotiations among the European Patent Office, the U.S. Patent Office, and the Japanese Patent Office; bilateral negotiations conducted by the U.S. Trade Representative between the United States and other individual nations; negotiations under the auspices of the World Intellectual Property Organization (WIPO), an agency of the United Nations, which is seeking to formulate a harmonization treaty; and negotiations in connection with the Uruguay round of the General Agreement on Tariffs and Trade (GATT), which sees intellectual property protection as an aspect of trade policy.

In the United States, the subject matter for patent protection is, by statute, any machine, article of manufacture, process, or composition of matter which meets the criteria of being new, useful, and nonobvious.

To some extent, these are terms of art. "Machine" and "article of manufacture" seem self-explanatory; however, "process" is designed to include only processes that involve, at some point, manipulation of physical entities. Processes that involve *only* mental steps cannot be subjects of patent protection. The advent of computer technology has somewhat muddied these waters, and it appears that courts are moving more and more toward accepting the protectability of processes that are essentially algorithms, at least in their inventive aspects. "Composition of matter" as the subject of patent protection is of high economic importance; the availability of patent protection for chemical compounds has been of tremendous value to the pharmaceutical industry. It may not be so intuitively obvious that "composition of matter" also includes altered organisms, including not only microorganisms but also genetically modified plants and higher animals.

The trilogy of statutory criteria applied to the subject matter can also be troublesome. By "new" is meant that the subject matter *as claimed* did not previously exist either as described in a publication or in physical form. As many elements of genetic testing and manipulation exist in some form in nature, it is a matter of skill to claim them in a "new" embodiment. "Useful" also has a particular meaning. The "use" must be other than as an object of curiosity or further research. This does not mean that research tools have no use, as long as that use is defined. For example, the technique of polyacrylamide gel electrophoresis would meet the statutory criterion of "useful" even though its "use" is to analyze materials rather than as a direct consumer product. "Nonobvious" is inherently subject to individual judgment, although it is putatively evaluated by an "objective" test—i.e., whether the subject matter taken as a whole would have been obvious to a skilled artisan at the time the invention was made.

The only property right conferred by the patent statute in the claimed subject matter is the right to exclude others for a limited time period (17 years from the date of issue of a patent) from making, using, or selling the subject matter claimed in the issued patent. To do any or all of these without the permission of the patent owner would be an act of infringement, which the patent owner can have a court enjoin and/ or for which a court can award damages. These remedies are also available against those who induce others to infringe and who contribute to infringement—for example, by selling an article that can only be used in an infringing process.

In the United States, this right to exclude others is very close to absolute. The United States has no requirements that the patent owner work the invention or cause it to be worked. The patent owner can simply sit on the protected patent right for the 17-year period. There is no provision for compulsory licensing, available at least at some level in many other jurisdictions, wherein a patent owner, most commonly a patent owner who is not working the invention, may be forced to permit others to practice it in return for a royalty. There is also no statutory "research exemption" in the United States, except for activities carried out in order to secure regulatory approval. While courts have carved out a limited exemption for purely philosophical or *de minimis* use, it appears that almost any commercial taint will be sufficient to remove the exemption. What is clear is that the alleged infringer cannot be certain that he or she is within the exemption. For example, the use of a research technique in connection with the development of a new product, even if that product is unrelated to the invention per se, cannot be assured to fall within any exemption. Other jurisdictions have more specific exemptions for research, and the United States appears to be among the least charitable nations toward infringing activities that are not totally dissociated from a commercial purpose.

For example, the owner of a DNA probe patented as a composition of matter in the United States will be able to exclude others from making, using, or selling the DNA probe within the United States. The owner of a U.S. patent claiming a process for the conduct of the polymerase chain reaction (PCR) will be able to exclude others from practicing this technique within the United States and from selling equipment dedicated to the practice of this technique in the United States.

Both of these examples relate to subject matters that are amenable for use in research. As noted above, there is in theory a research exemption in the United States for purely philosophical uses. It is not clear whether there is an exemption for use of what is specifically designed as a research tool when employed as a research tool. Probably there is not. Thus, claims to a method to conduct PCR are technically infringed by many university laboratories. As a practical matter, these users will likely be left alone by the current assignee, since such use has little economic impact on the assignee. On the other hand, use of the PCR technique to develop a product by a commercial enterprise or by a university operating under the sponsorship of a commercial enterprise might attract some action by the assignee. The best known activity in this regard is the widespread licensing of the Cohen-Boyer patent on recombinant technology by Stanford University acting on behalf of itself and the University of California. By making the cost of licenses extremely reasonable, Stanford has persuaded well over a hundred companies to become nonexclusive licensees.

The right to exclude is just that—it does not include any kind of permission for the patentee to practice the invention. Such practice might be prohibited by virtue of a dominating patent issued to another, by a requirement for compliance with regulatory statutes, or, of course, by economic constraints.

In the United States, the original "owner" entitled to patent is the first to invent the subject matter. (In all other jurisdictions except the Philippines, it is the first inventor to file for patent.) Of course the original owner can be, and usually is, obligated to transfer ownership to others, such as an employer or other sponsor.

Protectable Aspects of Genetic Testing and Manipulation

Because the technology of genetic testing is relatively new, and because the process of obtaining patent protection takes some time, it is not yet entirely clear what kinds of patent protection will ultimately be available for the methods and materials involved in genetic testing and manipulation. However, it is possible to apply the principles of the patent statute to these technologies and arrive at some logical inferences.

Because present techniques of genetic testing sometimes involve specific hybridization of target DNA sequences to probes, which are themselves composed of DNA, protection of these probes has been widely sought and obtained. Newer methods involve the use of PCR, which requires primers—again, also composed of DNA. Protection has also been sought for primers in this way. Such probes and primers are oligomers of particular DNA sequences that hybridize specifically to nucleic acid regions to be tested. The probes and primers are, of course, compositions of matter and are therefore statutory subject matter. They are also new, since even if the DNA sequence that is contained in them resides also in a gene somewhere, it does not reside there in the form of a defined probe. Whether or not they are nonobvious will depend on what is already known about the nature of the target. Whether or not they are useful will depend on whether they can test what they are supposed to test.

Another subject matter area is related to techniques or processes that might be useful in the conduct of these tests. The most notable example is the polymerase chain reaction that is useful in some aspects of this testing. Patent protection has been obtained for this technique generally and is now controlled by Hoffman-LaRoche. The subject matter is a process (although there are also composition of matter patents directed to enzymes that are particularly useful PCR). The process is new; there seem to be no descriptions anywhere of the process having been conducted in the past, despite contentions to the contrary in *DuPont* v. *Cetus*, 19 U.S.P.Q.2d 1174 (N.D. Cal. 1990); and no one seems to have raised serious doubts that the technique is useful.

Another type of protection that might be sought in connection with genetic testing is related to overall approaches for running the test. For example, the concept of using certain sources for the genetic material, such as the amniotic fluid or the chorionic villi, could theoretically be protected as processes, although I do not know whether such protection has been sought.

Finally, similar materials and techniques useful in genetic therapy and manipulation, presumably part of the rationale for genetic testing in the first place, can also be protected. For example, one patent application, WO 91/10741, filed as an international application under the auspices of WIPO in conformance with the Patent Cooperation Treaty, describes the incorporation of a desired DNA into a yeast artificial chromosome (YAC) (which permits large fragments of DNA to be manipulated in cell division like genes contained on the cell's own chromosomes) and the transfer of the altered YACs into embryonic stem cells of mice. The transformed embryonic stem cells are used to generate chimeric mice by adding them back to the blastocyst stage of embryo formation and then reimplanting the embryo in a pseudopregnant mouse. The extent to which patent protection can be obtained for this generalized technique is unclear; however, in principle, this approach represents a patentable process.

What Makes Patent Protection for Genetic Engineering Different?

While aspects of genetic engineering, including testing and therapy, are subject to the same statutes as is other subject matter, the nature of the technology gives rise to some issues that may not necessarily show up in more traditional technologies. The following is a discussion of these issues.

Discovery vs. Invention, or "You Mean You Can Patent A Gene?"

As alluded to above in connection with probes, in a sense, patent protection is being sought where the unique feature of the invention is something that already exists in nature—namely, a particular DNA sequence. The DNA sequence itself is not new because it already exists. The fact that no one knew what it was does not make it novel. Therefore, a decade or so ago there was some concern that the relevant materials in connection with genetic engineering would not meet the statutory test for novelty and thus not be patentable subject matter. This has turned out not to be the case, based on some substantial precedent.

A subtext in all of this is the distinction, if any, between discovery and invention. Although it is common to say that "discoveries" cannot be patented, Article 8 of the U.S. Constitution actually uses this word. These have also apparently become terms of art, and the issue of invention versus discovery has arisen in other contexts as well, most prominently in the case of computer software. While it is said that one cannot patent "laws of nature," elucidation of such laws of nature can lead to results that are significant and may be protectable. But retrieving and analyzing the sequence of a gene that already exists is perceptibly different in quality, if not kind, from inventing a better mousetrap or designing a new chemical compound. The structure of the mousetrap or compound did not exist before; the gene sequence did.

Although the case law is sparse, perhaps the most relevant precedents are the patentability of vitamin B-12 (*Merck v. Olin Mathieson*, 116 U.S.P.Q. 484 [4th Cir. 1958]), and the prostaglandins (*In re Bergstrom*, 166 U.S.P.Q. 256 [C.C.P.A. 1970]). These too are compounds that are found in nature. However, as the court stated in *Merck* (116 U.S.P.Q. at 490), there is clear contribution to society in obtaining the purified form of the vitamin as opposed to a crude liver extract. Therefore, claiming the vitamin as a purified compound makes sense. Similarly, the prostaglandin in its natural milieu cannot be manipulated conveniently, while pure prostaglandin can be used as a medicament.

Similarly, patents directed to purified and isolated DNA that encodes proteins that occur in nature have been granted and upheld. Most notable are the patents directed to the genes encoding human erythropoietin and tissue plasminogen activation (tPA). Patents have also been granted for the purified and isolated forms of the resulting proteins, though the patent directed to erythropoietin has been invalidated on other grounds.

In general, it has been possible to obtain composition-of-matter patents on materials that exist in nature so long as they can be claimed in a *form* different from that in which they exist there. There are several common approaches. These include claiming materials in "purified and isolated" forms, in specifically abbreviated forms such as peptide fragments of longer proteins, and in recombinant forms or, more generically, in other than their natural contexts. For example, claims directed to probes that will have sequence lengths substantially shorter than the DNA molecules in which the relevant sequence is contained in nature alter the form of the subject matter. Naturally occurring sequences of DNA can be claimed as linked (sometimes referred to as "recombinant") to DNAs to which the DNA sequences of interest are not ordinarily linked or to other materials with which they are not naturally associated.

In summary, the thing that sets these compositions apart from those usually claimed in the past—i.e., new pharmaceutical or other chemical compounds—is that the chemical architecture actually of interest is not designed by the inventor but by nature. The inventor merely places the predetermined molecular architecture in a form that is useful. Depending on the composition, the molecular architecture could be used as a medicament, as a catalyst in a process where the conditions are critical, or as a probe or standard in genetic testing.

Methods of diagnosis and treatment that involve novel insights resulting in process steps that are new per se or are new in combination offer no unique problems. However, the claimed processes themselves are often quite old—the combination of steps involved in performance of restriction length polymorphism methods or methods to administer medicaments are themselves old, and the inventiveness is conferred on them by the nature of materials used in carrying them out. This has actually caused some real problems. The practice of the U.S. Patent and Trademark Office (PTO) of applying, in a somewhat inconsistent manner, the holding in *In re Durden,* 763 F.2d 1406, 226 U.S.P.Q. 359 (Fed. Cir. 1985), has caused considerable controversy. In that case, the applicant admitted that the claimed process was old and that only the starting materials and products were new. The Federal Circuit panel held that the patentability of the new materials did not confer patentability on an old process. Another panel attempted to bail itself out of this fairly inconvenient decision in *In re Pleuddemann*, 15 U.S.P.Q.2d 1738 (Fed. Cir. 1990), which seemed to confer patentability on method-of-use claims where the material to be used was new, as opposed to method-to-make claims where the product was new. The PTO recognized that many method-to-make claims could simply be rewritten as method-of-use claims and saw this as a distinction without a difference. The matter is still unresolved and has been the subject of attempts to remedy it by statute. There are now at least two cases on appeal seeking to clarify this matter.

The issue of process patentability is of some considerable significance: It is relatively rare that an actual new technique per se, such as PCR, is advanced, as compared to the number of new applications of analogous processes. Also, due to specific provisions in the patent and trademark statutes, only claims directed to processes have any extraterritorial effect.

These Techniques Permit Alteration of "God's Creatures"

It is ironic that the scientific philosophy of the continuity and relatedness of living systems thought to have originated in Darwin's ideas, and perhaps most dramatically supported by the results of modern biotechnology, feeds the concerns of some that manipulation of plants, and more particularly animals, is in some way an interference with divine creation. Perhaps when humans were considered quite separate from animals, and certainly from plants, modifications made in these beings would have been seen as neutral. But people who see no theological implications in altering the CO_2 content of the atmosphere by relentlessly driving automobiles or in upsetting the global ecology by destroying the rain forests somehow see sinister implications in genetic manipulation of living creatures. This is certainly reinforced by the affirmation, clearly demonstrated by recombinant technology, that all organisms, from the lowliest bacterium to the most divinely touched human, translate the same genetic code in much the same way to obtain the same answer.

The manipulation of plants does not seem to be as emotional an issue as the manipulation of animals. And, indeed, protection can be sought and obtained for genetically transformed plants. It is clear that in the United States, at least, genetically transformed plants are patentable subject matter (*Ex parte Hibberd*, 227 U.S.P.Q. 443 [BPAI 1985]). This is in addition to protection of asexual plant varieties, generally obtained by classical means, by plant patents and of seeds under the Plant Variety Protection Act. A few patents have issued to genetically altered higher plants, but the comparative difficulty in obtaining approval of plant applications has led some to believe that negative pressure is being applied to the U.S. Patent Office on plant patenting.

While genetic manipulation of plant cells has posed more technical problems than genetic manipulation of microbial or animal cells, the genetic manipulation of whole plants, in the end, seems to have had considerable success. For example, while techniques for antisense manipulation of gene expression in animals have floundered, it has been possible to produce fruits and vegetables that can be ripened at will using antisense techniques. The Food and Drug Administration has indicated there will be no special regulatory problems involved in marketing these plants, although this statement has raised some protest.

Genetically manipulated animals (excluding humans) have also been held to be patentable subject matter (*Ex parte Allen*, 2 U.S.P.Q.2d 1425 [BPAI 1987]). Although the *Allen* case involved oysters as subject matter, it established the policy of the U.S. Patent and Trademark Office that the holding of patentability of bacteria in *In re Chakrabarty*, 197 U.S.P.Q. 72 (C.C.P.A. 1978), was controlling for multicellular as well as unicellular creatures. Although only one U.S. animal patent has issued (on the Harvard mouse as a cancer model system), there appears to be no theoretical reason why additional animal patents now pending will not issue as well. There has been some political pressure, however, to slow up the issuance of patents on animals for various reasons. It is believed by some that such manipulation is unethical; others are concerned about animal rights; and still others are concerned about their own economic interests.

It should also be noted that while human beings cannot be patented, techniques for manipulating them can. These techniques include genetic testing and therapy as well as traditional medical treatments. With respect to the exclusion of human beings as patentable subject matter, perhaps it should be recalled that intellectual property rights in a particular composition of matter, e.g., a human being, neither confers total ownership of the human being on the patent owner nor permits the patent owner to do anything in particular with the human being. It merely permits the patent owner to exclude *anyone else* from making, using, or selling this human being in the United States for the statutory period. Perhaps this could be interpreted as restricting the ability of the patented human to get a job. In any event, there appears to be no serious constituency advocating the inclusion of human beings within the ambit of statutory subject matter; the subject is mentioned here only because it seems interesting that so reflexive a distinction is drawn within the animal kingdom.

Biotechnology/Genetic Engineering Patents Affect Peculiar Sections of the Economy

By their very nature, biotechnology and genetic engineering are part and parcel of those sections of the economy that are most intimately connected with the average citizen—agriculture and health care. Because every individual is affected at the most basic level by the manner in which these sectors are managed, and because the nexus between the output of these sectors and the welfare of the individual is apparent to all, the effect of patents in this arena has an emotional appeal that would be lacking in industries whose impact is somewhat more remote or obscure. Even the highly publicized plight of the inventor of the intermittent windshield wiper, assertedly cheated at the hands of every automobile manufacturer, cannot generate the intensity of response attributable to patents that impact such familiar figures as farmers, doctors, nurses, and patients.

Because of the power of genetic testing and manipulation to affect agricultural products, an identifiable economic interest is at stake in the intellectual property rights associated with this subject matter. Farmers really are in a unique and transitional position. Even a casual observer can see that the infrastructure of agriculture has changed dramatically over the last one hundred years. Agriculture is becoming simply another industrialized and corporate sector of the economy, and this transition is happening while the romantic traditions of the family farm still exist in living memory.

The patent system is certainly designed to encourage the investment of capital, cooperative research, and the manipulation of the resulting technologies in a business environment. Farming is no exception. It cannot be denied that affording intellectual property protection to genetically transformed livestock will provide another mechanism that moves the conduct of agriculture farther away from an individual or small farmer. The questions are whether this effect is per se undesirable and whether the effect is of sufficient magnitude to make any difference. Other forces at work in the economy have had a much more drastic effect, including all technologically based improvements in agricultural efficiency that require capital investment to take advantage of them. Certainly it is not clear at this point to what extent special concessions should be made to farmers regarding what they might do with patented animals. Perhaps the Plant Variety Protection Act might be used as an example of how such exceptions could be carved out.

The other sector of the economy specifically impacted by genetic testing and therapy is the medical establishment. This seems to be a bit of a sleeper. The pharmaceutical industry has used the patent system very successfully since the end of World War II. However, over this same period the plethora of additional techniques, the availability of high technology "fixes," and the increased involvement of third-party payers continues to build the pressure for restructuring this system.

The United States is one of the few countries in the world that allows medical procedures to be patented. Many countries, especially in the Third World, do not even permit pharmaceuticals to be patented. It can

191

legitimately be questioned whether or not the patent protection of these subject matters is desirable.

The purpose of the patent system in these contexts is presumably to permit the considerable costs of research to be recovered through charging higher prices. In the case of pharmaceuticals, this purpose may have overextended itself and has probably permitted considerably more than the costs of research to be recovered. As medical costs continue to consume a larger and larger share of our gross national product, one might question whether the United States will find itself more squarely in the camp of the Third World and limit or deny patent protection for medicines and medical techniques. The political clout of pharmaceutical corporations is great, but recently voices have been raised objecting to the escalation of the prices charged for pharmaceuticals and openly suggesting that these prices constitute an abuse of the patent system.

Heavy Involvement by Academia in Genetic Manipulation

One of the major features of the biotechnology revolution has been the significant contribution of universities and nonprofit research institutes to the development of the technology. These institutions are putatively populated by individuals whose interests have been more focused on scientific glory, professional recognition, and academic success than on recovery of investment or profit making. While some have defected to more lucrative fields once the opportunity became clear, pressures still remain in the academic establishment to advance the cause of research independent of economic considerations.

Perhaps the most notable example of the perception that noncommercial institutions are expanding their potential commercial horizons to an undesirable level is the current furor over the filing of patent applications covering well over two thousand DNA sequences identified as novel in a cDNA library recovered by reverse transcription from the human brain at the National Institutes of Health (NIH). The application as filed abroad is published as PCT application WO93/00353. While there was no particular complaint about the one-by-one patenting of genes encoding particular proteins upon recovery and sequencing of these segments of DNA, the remarkable efficiency with which thousands of unique DNA sequences, presumably from the most significant portions of the genome, have been recovered has made a fair number of people nervous. It will be recalled that the human genome is thought to contain about 100,000 genes; these occupy only about 1 percent of the genome. The rest is presumably nonsense, according to current dogma. Since the sequences were recovered from genes in the process of translation, these sequences are thought to be associated with the relevant 1 percent.

Many of the arguments advanced in support of the notion that NIH is out of line in attempting to patent this plethora of sequences have rested on legal considerations independent of the origin of the invention. However, the origin of the invention has been a factor in motivating these arguments. It has been claimed that the attempt to obtain protection for these sequences undermines the atmosphere of international cooperation originally associated with the Human Genome Project. Also, because it concerned a government invention, the application for patent saw the light of day very early in its career. Had application been made by a private company, no one would have known about it, presumably, until a foreign counterpart had been published some 18 months later. (This assumes the usual scenario, wherein the private company files first in the U.S., does not itself disclose the fact of its filing, and files abroad within the Convention year to obtain the priority (benefit of the filing date) of the U.S. application in other countries. While U.S. applications are secret until issued as patents, foreign applications are published 18 months from their priority dates, according to standard statutory procedures in non-U.S. jurisdictions.) No one would question the *policy* behind a commercial enterprise applying for a patent of this type; the policy of NIH has been questioned vociferously. In short, while legal arguments such as those in the following paragraph have been marshaled in support of the idea that NIH is somehow unjustified in making this application, the furor has arisen, in my view, because of the high profile and perceived role of NIH. It is now known that at least two private companies have filed similar applications; this seems to be stirring relatively little controversy.

Legal arguments include the assertion that the NIH application distorts the intent that inventions to be patented must be "useful." The NIH claims are directed to a collection of DNA segments, some of which are associated with genes of known biological function and others not. It has been argued that the important decision on the meaning of statutory utility (*Brenner* v. *Manson*, 383 U.S. 519, 148 U.S.P.Q. 689 [1966]) mandates that only the type of utility associated with segments of genes of known biological function meets the requirements of the statute. Another argument independent of the NIH origin of the application is that the invention is obvious since anyone of ordinary skill could obtain the sequences claimed using standard, commercially available, and very powerful robotic techniques. However, other arguments are directly related to the origins of the application as coming from a government laboratory for which patent protection is potentially inappropriate.

To some extent, the policy arguments may become academic, since the inventor of the claimed DNA, Dr.Craig Venter, has left NIH to head The Genomic Research Institute (TIGR), a foundation funded by a private company, Human Genome Sciences, which proposes to commercialize the results of continued sequencing activities on the part of the foundation. If NIH abandons its own application, the inventor may have to be offered ownership of those sequences already obtained.

A major concern with regard to the NIH application focuses simply on the apparently sudden realization that there are "business" concerns being addressed by what was supposed to be a purely intellectual endeavor. Fears have been expressed that, by framing the results of the genome sequencing project in a business context, competitiveness will replace cooperation in the project, and scientific progress will be slowed.

Policy Issues

According to the U.S. Constitution, the patent system is supposed to "promote the progress of science and the useful arts by securing for limited times to (authors and) inventors the exclusive right to their (respective writings and) discoveries" (Article 8). It is not clear how the framers of the Constitution envisioned this limited monopoly as promoting progress. But it is clear how the current operation of the patent system does this.

For one thing, the patent system seems to provide sufficient confidence for established companies to engage in research and development, with the knowledge that they will be able to price the products of that research without fear of competition. For the multiplicity of young companies forming around particular aspects of biotechnology in the last 10 or 15 years (including companies grounded in particular techniques of genetic therapy and genetic testing), the availability of patent protection appears to provide sufficient confidence for investors that the considerable start-up, development, and regulatory clearance costs involved in bringing these technologies to market will be recovered eventually. This is important because the inventions relevant to genetic testing and manipulation are not available through tinkering in the garage. The significant manner in which the patent system promotes the progress of science and the useful arts in this context is by directing the flow of money into fairly large-scale research projects that are expected to yield significant results.

The flip side of this is that the various research programs are not operated in vacuums; the products they produce are interrelated. The exclusivity conferred on company A as a result of its research efforts may prevent the development of additional products by company B or institution C because some intermediate step is not available to B or C without a license from company A. Company A, as stated above, is in no way obligated under the U.S. system to provide such a license. There is, however, a statutory exception with respect to work devoted to securing regulatory approval for drugs or medical devices in preparation for their sale after the patent expires (35 U.S.C. §271[e]).

The double-edged sword of encouraging research but failing to require allowance of its use by others raises a number of policy issues.

Is the Patent System Necessary to Maintain U.S. Competitiveness?

There is a school of thought that maintenance of a strong intellectual property system whenever technology is made, used, or sold is necessary for the United States to maintain its lead in one of the very few technologies in which it is still considered to have a lead, namely, biotechnology. The position of the United States has been to insist that others maintain strong intellectual property systems applicable to pharmaceuticals and biotechnology.

There is some question whether this perception is correct. The availability of patent protection has clearly encouraged investors over the last decade. Clearly the availability of patents has encouraged pharmaceutical houses to maintain research programs. But whether this system will favor U.S. industry at the expense of foreign applicants is not so clear. Under the Paris Convention, foreign applicants also have access to this system of protection. There is increasing pressure for the United States to get rid of those few provisions of the patent statute that are prejudicial to foreign applicants—e.g., provisions favoring U.S. applicants in priority contests for the first-to-invent claimed subject matter.

Indeed the most serious inequities with respect to foreign inventors arise out of the first-to-invent system where, in contrast to "first-inventor-to-file" systems, invention prior to filing may be shown. However, except for an application filed abroad itself, for which priority is claimed, all activities in proof must have been conducted in the United States! Thus, in comparison with U.S. firms, companies conducting research abroad are at a disadvantage in obtaining U.S. patents. The earliest possible date they can establish, assuming that their research is in fact conducted outside the United States, is the filing date of their priority application. The company conducting research within the United States, on the other hand, would be able to adduce evidence, if needed, in support of an earlier conception of the invention followed by a diligent effort to reduce to practice—all within the United States. Whether the first-to-invent system operates to favor U.S. technology, absent these provisions that stack the cards in favor of U.S. inventors, becomes an open question.

A counterforce in this respect is found in the one-year grace period (actually a statutory bar) provided to applicants for patent in the United States. This has the result that when, for example, publication has occurred, patent production can often be obtained in the United States, but only in a few other jurisdictions (Japan has a six-month grace period, Canada has a one-year grace period, Europe has none). A case in point is the Cohen-Boyer patent on genetic engineering, which could be obtained only in the United States because of intervening publications that precluded its patenting elsewhere (except Canada). Thus, companies conducting research using these techniques in the United States are obligated to take a license, while those practicing the same techniques abroad are not.

Is the Patent System of Reward Legitimate for the Health Care Industry?

The desired effect of the patent system in the United States to promote progress operates essentially through a business mechanism, providing monetary rewards if the results of scientific progress are commercially successful. One might question whether the patent system as an adjunct to the free market economy is suitably applicable to health care or whether health care, including genetic testing, genetic therapy, and so forth, is not a responsibility of society as a whole, in which case commercialization is out of place.

There may be other ways to encourage research in medicine. There are squadrons of people who work very hard at promoting the progress of science simply for the intellectual satisfaction involved in it and in return for reasonable financial support and recognition. The universities and research institutions are full of them. Perhaps a more reasonable way to encourage research in health care would be to expand the funding for such institutions and to educate people to take satisfaction and to admire achievement unrelated to financial gain.

Similarly, despite the well-known prevalence of subsidies, agriculture has generally been thought to be a legitimate profit-making enterprise that operates like any other participant in the capitalist system. Agriculture absent the profit motive does not seem to have worked well, although the reasons for this are not clear.

Does the Intellectual Property System Widen the Gap Between Rich and Poor?

One of the effects of the increasingly deregulated free market economy where financial incentives have become more and more important has been to widen the gap between technologically or otherwise highly trained and educated individuals and those who are not. It may be that the patent system, because it fits so well into capital investment, large-scale research projects, and fostering of technology in general, which in turn promotes larger scale enterprises and the need for capital investment, moves society in a direction where increasing numbers of people will be unable to compete successfully. Consideration should be given to whether this result is real and in any way attributable to the intellectual property system.

Should the Intellectual Property System or Any Other System Be Used to Encourage This Technology?

There is a substantial element of society that is resistant to the advancement of the ability to manipulate animals genetically and humans especially. To the extent that the intellectual property protection system encourages the continuation of research, which permits ever more powerful techniques to control human physiology, and therefore to some extent human behavior, such protection is desirable only to the extent that the increased ability to perform such manipulations is considered desirable. Much mockery is made of the "Luddite" attitudes of those who contend that the ability of people to control the fate of the earth is not necessarily something that should be encouraged. Most of this mockery is based on the present reality that the ultimate devastating catastrophe has not yet happened. After all, people still exist here, many of them living pretty good lives. But the fact that others have cried wolf before does not mean that the wolf is not at the door now. Perhaps some consideration should be given to the logical conclusions of activities in which we are presently engaged, such as encouraging the overpopulation of the earth and demanding ever more of earth's resources.

Should the Research Exemption Be Codified and Made Explicit?

The converse of the foregoing section is that the patent system creates obstacles to conducting further research. If the previous section is to be believed, this might be a desirable result; however, there are many who would be direct or indirect beneficiaries of research who think otherwise. One approach to limiting this perceived downside would be to create a statutory research exemption. In effect, in the United States, one such exemption has been created already—35 U.S.C. §271(e), which exempts research directed to obtaining regulatory approval. The courts are in the process of interpreting this statutory section, and it appears, despite its seemingly limited scope, this section casts a fairly broad net and may significantly protect certain organizations using patented techniques in research or development of a specific product. This level of protection for research may be all that is needed, provided nonregulated industries could also be included. Researchers not involved in product development are fairly safe anyway, since there appears to be little point in enjoining infringers or collecting damages if there is no profit involved.

Nevertheless, there is some argument that a research exemption should be clarified and conformed more closely to that available in other jurisdictions. Specifically, use of the patented subject matter for a purpose other than infringing commercial activity would be permitted. This is actually the converse of the exemption created by 35 U.S.C. §271(e).

Conclusion

The availability of intellectual property protection for compositions and processes related to genetic testing and manipulation leads to consequences at a number of levels that affect the amount of effort put into research, the manner in which the economic system will structure itself, and the attitudes of the public and the professionals involved toward various ethical issues. The result of these consequences will have a significant impact on the nature of society, and, ultimately, global ecology. With issues of this scope, the threshold issue is, perhaps, the extent to which intellectual property protection for such compositions and methods is desirable. In other words, should limitations be placed on the extent of intellectual property protection as a matter of public policy?

Assuming that it is desirable to have *some* system for intellectual property protection remain in place for compositions and processes related to genetic testing and manipulation, attention can be directed to how to best arrange this system to achieve the greatest good. Can the subject matter definitions in the statute be designed to encourage only those types of inventions that seem to offer some help to society? What kinds of inventions are these? Should the system be reoriented in order to more easily protect mental processes reflected in real-world manipulations, where those mental processes really constitute the invention? Should the bases for finding sufficient utility to satisfy the statutory requirement be strengthened or weakened? Should certain sectors of the economy be excluded from the sphere in which exclusivity is granted? After all, patent rights are, at this time, territorial; should there also be "field-of-use" restrictions? Finally, should specific legislation that merely tinkers with the existent patent system be considered? One example is a bill that would provide patent protection for otherwise unpatentable processes under certain specified conditions, designed to reverse the *Durden* decision mentioned previously. This would provide an added extraterritorial effect to the relevant patent in which a process claim might not otherwise issue, due to provisions unique to process claims in the patent statute as provided in the 1988 trade bill.

The questions related to simply modifying the system itself are in essence less global but easier to tackle, and the answers have a far greater chance of resulting in implementation. In the final analysis, the global questions and the more limited policy considerations are intertwined, and perhaps it is artificial to separate them.

10

Intellectual Property and Genetic Testing: A Commentary

Thomas J. White, Ph.D.

The four sections of Kate Murashige's article can be examined in the context of the issues surrounding the patent application filed by the National Institutes of Health on several thousand complementary DNA clone sequences. Critics of this policy have argued that the sequences should not be patentable because they are incomplete, have no known function, and are not useful. Another concern is that the decision to file might inhibit international collaborations on the Human Genome Project, slow the exchange of sequence data among scientists, and overwhelm patent offices and examiners. Supporters of the NIH action have justified the filing by claiming that such patents will aid the commercialization of new medical products while *not* filing will inhibit it. Opponents have maintained that just the opposite will occur (Adler 1992; Anderson 1992). All parties agree that a possible result may be extensive litigation and that the costs and time involved might be better spent on other social or medical needs.

Some of the uproar over the NIH action comes from scientists who are unfamiliar with the various types of patents, the criteria for obtaining a patent, and existing precedent based on issued U.S. patents and patents that have been held valid upon litigation. It is a common practice to file an initial patent application on incomplete sequences and subsequently add information in later versions, called a "continuation-in-part" (White et al. 1990). This practice may permit the inventor to obtain an issued claim on a complete gene sequence while retaining the original filing date of the first application. It also allows scientists who make subsequent inventive contributions to a patent application to receive "credit," thereby addressing a concern raised in Chapter 11 by Joan Overhauser. Such a strategy was used for the Factor VIII gene (Scandella et al. 1992; Houghton et al. 1989; Toole and Fritsch 1988). So completeness, per se, has not been an absolute criterion for filing or patentability. However, few of these patents have been litigated, so the success of this strategy in yielding valid, enforceable patent claims is largely untested.

A similar situation applies for genes or sequences of unknown function. For example, what is the biological "function" of the VNTR (variable number of tandem repeat) locus patented by Ray White at the University of Utah (White et al. 1990)? Similarly, the probe fragment patented by Walter Bodmer (a former director of HUGO) that serves as a marker for familial adenomatous polyposis has no known function (Bodmer et al. 1992). Finally, the functions of *mcf* transforming genes and of the K-*ras* oncogene (as a GTPase signal to an effector protein) were unknown when the Cold Spring Harbor Laboratories and the State University of New York (SUNY), respectively, filed patent applications on these sequences (Wigler 1989; Perucho et al. 1988). Although these individuals and institutions may be justifiably concerned about the NIH patent filings, these are clear exceptions to the requirement to know a gene's function before a patent application is filed or granted.

There is also some confusion over the definition of "use." For example, the medical utility of *ras* probes was mainly theoretical at the time the SUNY patent application was filed (and allowed). Although the *ras* protooncogenes are mutated in many types of cancers, the mere detection of mutant *ras* in a lung cell is not predictive of disease stage, prognosis, or response to treatment. Analogously, what is the certain "use" of detecting the types of human papillomavirus that are associated with cervical cancer if only a small fraction of women infected with the high-risk types actually progress to disease? Arguments can be made for a *likely* use, such as in the identification of a subset of women at higher risk (Morris and Nightingale 1988), but how much proof of utility is required at the time of filing and during prosecution of the patent application? By listing these examples of issued patents on gene sequences that are partial and have unknown function and speculative utility, one is not arguing for patenting of partial cDNA clones but rather pointing out that several of the arguments against patenting them have not prevented similar patents from being granted. Interestingly, some of the most vocal critics of the NIH action have obtained patents that do not meet the standards now being advocated.

To address the question regarding the benefit to society and medicine of gene patents, one can easily enumerate many medical products that have resulted from biotechnology in the past 15 years. Figure 1 illustrates 10 recombinant drugs or vaccines that are currently marketed and for which patents have been granted (Carbonare 1991). The length of the bars indicates the development time between a

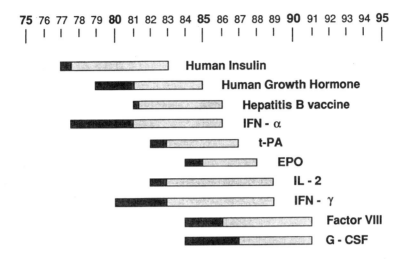

Figure 1. Development of biotechnical pharmaceuticals. Carbonare, B.D., "Recombinant Proteins Used in Medicine." *Genetic Engineering: What's Happening at Roche?* Basel, Switzerland: F. Hoffmann-La Roche, Inc., p. 19. Copyright © 1991.

technical breakthrough, such as purification of the natural protein or cloning of its gene, through the preclinical and clinical test phases (dark and light shading, respectively) to launch of the product. Not only have these products been patented, but to my knowledge there is no example of an approved recombinant therapeutic that has *not* been patented. In the absence of a likelihood that a patent will be granted, companies are reluctant to make the considerable investment necessary to win drug approval. Patents on closely related sequences or compositions filed by several companies may be the subject of an "interference" action (e.g., in the case of patent applications on interferon alpha and granulocyte-macrophage colony stimulating factor). Prior to the resolution of the interference action, companies sometimes negotiate cross-licensing agreements so that more than one can market the product, and the ultimate interference loser pays royalties to the company that prevails.

However much one accepts or rejects the above arguments for patenting genes for potential medicines, there is also a contrasting list of important genetic compositions and processes for which patents were not sought. Many of these have been of great benefit to research, medicine, and society and were commercialized despite the lack of patent protection. Foremost among such genes and proteins are the commercially successful restriction enzymes that laid the foundation for recombinant DNA techniques. The cost of developing a new native or cloned enzyme, however, is two orders of magnitude below that of developing a new drug. Also, other unrelated restriction enzymes with a similar or identical cleavage specificity can be found that would relatively quickly render a composition patent valueless. Nevertheless, restriction enzymes are a counterexample to the argument that the lack of patent protection, per se, is a bar to developing a commercially successful recombinant product.

Important processes that were not patented include those for making monoclonal antibodies, the Southern blot procedure, and the two main DNA sequencing techniques. All these processes are widely used in products and services and are commercialized because ways have been found to provide value despite widespread competition. This is analogous to improvements in surgical and radiological techniques and may anticipate how advances in the delivery of somatic gene therapy may be implemented.

On the other hand, patenting of processes also need not inhibit basic and applied research. The "Cohen and Boyer" patent (Cohen and Boyer 1980) on recombinant DNA techniques has certainly not impeded their adoption; the "Jeffreys" patent (Jeffreys 1986) on DNA fingerprinting has been commercialized through licensing for criminal forensic applications; and the polymerase chain reaction (PCR) patents issued to Cetus Corporation (Mullis et al. 1990, 1987; Mullis 1987) did not inhibit the extensive proliferation of this technique for research in academic institutions. For example, PCR is used in every phase of the Human Genome Project for the storage and recovery of sequence information through sequence-tagged sites, genetic mapping, physical mapping, mutation analysis, and sequence analysis. Other recently issued U.S. patents on processes such as the RAPD technique (randomly amplified polymorphic DNA) (Livak et al. 1992; Hartley 1991) or NASBA (nucleic acid sequence based amplification) (Malek et al. 1992) will generate similar issues. There are also many pending patents on techniques that may be widely used, such as immunoglobulin combinatorial libraries (Orlandi et al. 1989) and selective evolution of ligands by exponential enrichment (Tuerk and Gold 1990).

With this brief introduction to existing precedent on patents for genes and processes, what might represent a biotechnology industry perspective? First, there is no industrywide consensus on many of these issues, and there are specific disagreements among the various trade associations, large pharmaceutical corporations, and entrepreneurial firms. Second, it may be useful to distinguish between the value of patents for therapeutics and for diagnostics because of the great difference in their respective development costs. With these qualifications in mind, the conventional wisdom is that for recombinant drugs and vaccines, the likelihood of obtaining patents on compositions of matter, processes, and uses is essential in making the decision to invest in research and development and in recovering the costs of clinical testing and drug registration. Furthermore, exclusive rights for the life of the patents are required for the same reasons. To some extent, wider access to a drug by other firms would be available through cooperative cross-licensing of products—a common practice in the pharmaceutical industry.

In diagnostic applications of genetic technology, composition-of-matter patents are important, but since many of the genes for genetic disorders will be cloned at academic institutions, it is likely that nonexclusive licenses will be granted (e.g., for cystic fibrosis gene sequences). However, process patents, such as those for PCR and the pending applications for ligase chain reaction (LCR) (Barany 1991; Richards and Jones 1989), are likely to become increasingly important. *Use* patents may be of little value inasmuch as the ultimate potential infringers are the patients/customers. For example, if the commercial "use" of a genetic marker is for forensic testing, it might be difficult to prevent a purchaser from using the same product for determining paternity or for tissue typing for bone marrow transplantation or monitoring for engraftment. However, a patent gives its owner certain rights over a competitor who induces or contributes to infringement.

The increase in patenting of genes, processes, and uses has led many academic scientists to question whether their normal research activities constitute patent infringement or whether these fall under an "experimental use" exception. This refers to a judicially created exception to the normal definition of an infringer as anyone who "without authority makes, uses, or sells any patented invention, within the United States during the term of the patent. . ." (35 U.S.C. §271 (1988). Karp (1991) has reviewed the history of the exception and the policy justifications that counsel against broadening its application and has provided some compromise recommendations on limited experimental use. Although this subject is too complex to analyze in detail in this commentary, in simple terms a "research exception" is narrowly defined to be applicable only where the patented technology is used to verify the claims of the patent or for experiments that are "simply philosophical" in nature. A key consideration is whether the activity in question deprives the owner of the patent of something to which he or she is entitled. For example, the use of a patented enzyme for its intended and identified purpose (e.g., in PCR or LCR) would not qualify for the exception merely because it is used in a university. A "simple philosophical" inquiry in this context might include measurements of an enzyme's kinetic characteristics or a determination of its crystal structure, but not an experiment that itself might become the basis for obtaining government funding, filing patent applications, or pursuing other legitimate interests of the academic institution.

With these unresolved issues being actively debated, it may be instructive to consider the impact of some of the proposals for changes in policy on gene patents. Although it is clear that partial sequences have been patented, perhaps this could be restricted from now on. However, the consequences might be worse than the problem. Partial clones are already widely published long before complete genomic sequences are obtained and characterized or, alternatively, spliced mRNA transcripts isolated and understood. Thus, patenting of partial sequences encourages publication as opposed to suppression of the information as a trade secret until all possible cDNA and genomic clones of multiple gene families are obtained. In the United States, a patent application can still be filed up to a year *after* publication, so the argument that filing inherently inhibits publication is not necessarily the case.

The notion that genes of unknown function should not be patentable also has foreseeable deleterious consequences for research. Many potentially useful genes have no known function; besides, must an inventor wait until one or *all* functions are known? For example, the polyfunctional cytokine leukemia inhibitory factor has at least a dozen activities (Heath 1992). How do we define the "function" of lactate dehydrogenase: as a metabolic enzyme (Wistow et al. 1990) or as a crystallin lens protein? Such a policy might actually discourage research on medically beneficial genes that have no known function. It also confuses biological function with the legal requirement for utility. Thus, the *function* of alpha-one antitrypsin is as a protease inhibitor, but its medical *use* might be as a treatment for emphysema.

Another proposed policy change is to allow patents only on the "uses" of genes. But can "use" be an educated guess, an in vitro activity, or must it be based on preclinical or even clinical efficacy results? If "use" were only defined and proven by the results of clinical trials, then those very results might not be published rapidly. Is the use of a polymorphic gene fragment simply as a genetic marker enough of a use to validate a patent claim? Although Kiley (1992) has argued for a "substantial" utility definition, his perspective is biased toward gene products used for therapeutics; yet one of the most commonly used forensic tests involves a partial gene of unknown function that has no other foreseeable use than as a polymorphic genetic marker (White et al. 1990). One could argue that as little information as knowing that a gene has two alleles could still be "useful," since it could exclude the possibility that certain criminal evidence could have been contributed by a particular suspect. Since most genes have two or more alleles, and it is hard to argue that avoiding a wrongful prosecution or reversing a conviction is not useful, it would seem that most partial gene sequences could still meet even this minimal "use" criterion for patentability as long as both the use and *how* to use it are demonstrated. As mentioned above, it can also be difficult to enforce *use* patents when a product sold for one purpose is used by a physician for another purpose. Finally, this strategy might inundate the U.S. Patent and Trademark Office (PTO) with a new application on every newly discovered use.

Currently, gene sequences are required to be deposited with the PTO but not in a publicly accessible database such as GenBank. If a sequence is deposited with GenBank, the depositor can temporarily restrict access until a scientific paper appears but cannot restrict access until after a patent issues. The date of public access to the sequence constitutes a publication that may bar others who might isolate an identical sequence from claiming it as novel. So one potential policy change would be for the PTO to require the deposit of a sequence in a public database at the time of filing of a patent application and to use this date as a definition of "first to file."

To some, patents have become the scapegoat for actions that are more a matter of policy over the direction and form that research and development may take. But policies are a matter of judgment and choice. For example, the University of California State Oath of Allegiance and Patent Agreement requires each employee "to assign inventions and patents to the university and to promptly report and fully disclose . . . potentially patentable inventions to [the university patent office]." An alternative choice could be for the university (or government) to require all gene sequences to be published. Medically valuable gene products could still be protected by process, use, and in some cases even composition-of-matter patents (*In re Anthony*, 162 U.S.P.Q. 594 (C.C.P.A. 1969); *In re Wiggins*, 158 U.S.P.Q. [C.C.P.A. 1968]). The university would thereby stick to its traditional primary purposes of instructing and gaining new knowledge for the public good but might forego some potential sources of financial support via licensing fees and royalties. This policy might be a more effective instrument for preventing undesirable developments in genome research than a policy that refuses to grant patents on partial genes.

Some of the points in Kate Murashige's chapter have been illustrated with examples that represent the current state of affairs on gene patenting and the possible impact of various policy changes. Patent applications on the partial cDNA clones may neither provide all the benefits the government hopes nor result in all the detrimental consequences opponents fear. That is, even if patents are awarded on partial clones, they will neither aid the patent licensee nor prevent others from obtaining patents on the complete clones, as Eisenberg (1992) has elegantly observed. Further, existing patents and publications may not even prevent a company from obtaining a patent on a new pharmaceutical composition for a known compound that previously had no practical therapeutic utility (*In re Anthony*, 162 U.S.P.Q. 594 (C.C.P.A. 1969);

In re Wiggins, 158 U.S.P.Q. [C.C.P.A. 1968]). If the NIH patent applications do not achieve their purpose, perhaps the time and money spent on them would be better applied to demonstrating the medical utility of the sequences or to other aspects of public health such as providing wider access to affordable health care.

Acknowledgments

Thanks are extended S. Sias, G. Gould, P. Rocha, J. Sninsky, T. Taforo, R. Cook-Deegan, M. Frankel, B. Epstein, and D. Gelfand for helpful comments on the manuscript. The opinions expressed in the article are solely those of the author.

References

Adler, R.G. 1992. "Genome Research: Fulfilling the Public's Expectations for Knowledge and Commercialization." *Science* 257:908–914.

Anderson, C. 1992. "IH Defends Gene Patents as Filing Deadline Approaches." *Nature* 357:270.

Barany, F. 1991. "Genetic Disease Detection and DNA Amplification Using Cloned Thermostable Ligase." *Proceedings of the National Academy of Science USA* 88:189–193.

Bodmer, W.F., Murday, V.A., Bailey, C.J., and Williamson, R., Inventors. U.S. Patent #5,098,823. Chromosome-specific nucleic acid probe for familial polyposis coli. Filed: August 11, 1988. Issued: March 24, 1992.

Carbonare, B.D. 1991. "Recombinant Proteins Used in Medicine." *Genetic Engineering: What's Happening at Roche?* Basel, Switzerland: F. Hoffmann-La Roche, Inc.

Cohen, S.N. and Boyer, H.W., Inventors. U.S. Patent #4,237,224. Process for producing biologically functional molecular chimeras. Filed: January 4, 1979. Issued: December 2, 1980.

Eisenberg, R.S. 1992. "Genes, Patents and Product Development." *Science* 257:903–908.

Hartley, J.L., Inventor. U.S. Patent #5,043,272. Amplification of nucleic acid sequences using oligonucleotides of random sequence as primers. Filed: April 27, 1989. Issued: August 27, 1991.

Heath, J.K. 1992. "Can There Be Life With LIF?" *Nature* 359:17.

Houghton, M., Choo, Q.-L., and Kuo, G., Inventors. U.K. Patent Application GB #2,212,511. Hepatitis C Virus. Filed: November 18, 1988. Date of Publication: July 26, 1989.

Jeffreys, A.J., Inventor. U.K. Patent Application #2,166,445. Polynucleotide probes. Filed: October 14, 1985. Date of Publication: May 8, 1986.

Karp, J.P. 1991. "Experimental Use as Patent Infringement: The Impropriety of a Broad Exception." *Yale Law Journal* 100:2169–2188.

Kiley, T.D. 1992. "Patents on Random Complementary DNA Fragments?" *Science* 257:915–918.

Livak, K.J., Rafalski, J.A., Tingey, S.V, and Williams, J.G., Inventors. U.S. Patent #5,126,239. Process for detecting polymorphisms on the basis of nucleotide differences. Filed: March 14, 1990. Issued: June 30, 1992.

Malek, L.T., Davey, C., Henderson, G., Sooknanan, R., Inventors. U.S. Patent #5,130,238. Enhanced nucleic acid amplification process. Filed: August 23, 1989. Issued: July 14, 1992.

Morris, B.J. and Nightingale, B., Inventors. International Publication Number WO88/06634. A method of detection of carcinogenic human papillomavirus. Filed: February 24, 1988. International Publication Date: September 7, 1988.

Mullis, K.B., Inventor. U.S. Patent #4,683,202. Process for amplifying nucleic acid sequences. Filed: October 25, 1985. Issued: July 28, 1987.

Mullis, K.B., Erlich, H.A., Arnheim, N., Horn, G.T., Saiki, R.K., Scharf, S.J., Inventors. U.S. Patent #4,683,195. Process for amplifying nucleic acid sequences. Filed: February 7, 1986. Issued: July 28, 1987.

Mullis, K.B., Erlich, H.A., Gelfand, D.H., Horn, G.T., and Saiki, R.K., Inventors. U.S. Patent #4,965,188. Process for amplifying, detecting and/or cloning nucleic acid sequences using a thermostable enzyme. Filed: June 17, 1987. Issued: October 23, 1990.

Orlandi, R., Gussow, D.H., Jones, P.T., and Winter, G. 1989. "Cloning Immunoglobulin Variable Domains for Expression by the Polymerase Chain Reaction." *Proceedings of the National Academy of Science USA* 86:3833–3837.

Perucho, M., Nakamoto, H., and Yamamoto, F., Inventors. U.S. Patent #4,725,550. Novel mutation of the C-K-*ras* oncogene activated in a human lung carcinoma. Filed: January 19, 1984. Issued: February 16, 1988.

Richards, R.M. and Jones, T., Inventors. International Publication Number WO89/12696. Method and reagents for detecting nucleic acid sequences. Filed: June 16, 1989. International Publication Date: December 28, 1989.

Scandella, D.H., Drohan, W.N., Zimmerman, T.S., and Fulcher, C.A., Inventors. U.S. Patent #5,149,637. Recombinant factor VIIIC fragments. Filed: September 20, 1990. Issued: September 22, 1992.

Toole, J.J., Jr., and Fritsch, E., Inventors. U.S. Patent #4,757,006. Human Factor VIII: c gene and recombinant methods for production. Filed: October 28, 1983. Issued: July 12, 1988.

Tuerk, C. and Gold, L. 1990. "Systematic Evolution of Ligands by Exponential Enrichment: RNA Ligands to Bacteriophage T4 DNA Polymerase." *Science* 249:505–510.

White, R.L., Nakamura, Y., O'Connell, P., and Leppert, M.F., Inventors. U.S. Patent #4,963,663. Genetic identification employing DNA probes of variable number tandem repeat loci. Filed: February 18, 1989. Issued: October 16, 1990.

Wigler, M., Inventor. U.S. Patent #4,866,166. Bioassay for transforming genes and genes detected thereby. Filed: August 31, 1984. Issued: September 12, 1989.

Wistow, G., Anderson, A., and Piatigorsky, J. 1990. "Evidence for Neutral and Selective Processes in the Recruitment of Enzyme-Crystallins in Avian Lenses." *Proceedings of the National Academy of Science USA* 87:6277–6280.

11

Intellectual Property and Genetic Testing: A Scientist's Perspective

Joan Overhauser, Ph.D.

To discuss the patentability of DNA sequences that are involved in genetic testing, it is important to keep in mind what the United States defines as patentable material. Two legal requirements must be met: (1) the subject matter for patent protection must be any machine, article of manufacture, process, or composition of matter; and (2) it must be new, useful, and nonobvious. There is no argument that DNA sequences are a composition of matter, a fulfillment of the first requirement, and according to the interpretation of the law by patent lawyers, they are new since they are not present as a separate DNA sequence. Thus, from a legal standpoint, DNA sequences fulfill the requirements for patentable material. And there is already precedence for the patenting of DNA sequences.

When one thinks of patents, it is usual to associate them with an invention, "a product of the imagination" according to Webster's dictionary. From a scientist's perspective, DNA sequences are not a product of the imagination but a code that predates the inception of the experiment. A major area of research in recent years has been in the identification of specific DNA sequences from the 3×10^9 base pairs that code for the genes that are involved in human disease. The importance of this work is that once a disease gene has been identified and sequenced, genetic screening can be performed to inform individuals of their risk of having a disease or of having children with the disease. Another consequence of the identification of the disease gene is that it can lead to an enhanced understanding of the mechanism of the disease, which can lead to therapies that reduce the clinical severity of the disease or extend the life of the affected individual.

The topic of patentability has gained attention in the scientific community with the filing of patents for over two thousand partial cDNA sequences whose protein function is presently unknown. There are several issues that need to be addressed:

1. Should DNA sequences be patentable?

2. Will the issuance of patents inhibit research?

3. If DNA sequences are patented, who should obtain the rights?

Should DNA Sequences Be Patentable?

One extreme is to say no, that no patents based on DNA sequences should be issued. Although several patents have already been issued for DNA sequences, this should not prevent the reevaluation of patentability of such material as scientific and ethical issues are raised.

An intermediate solution would be that the entire DNA sequence of a gene must be known and the biologic function of the protein determined prior to consideration of a patent application. The gene for cystic fibrosis may fit that category, since its DNA sequence as well as the function of the coded protein have been determined. Because of the high incidence of cystic fibrosis carriers in the general population, it is clear that testing individuals who may be at risk for having children with the disease and developing gene therapy for those affected will be an active area of research that may deserve patent protection.

The other extreme would be the patenting of any DNA sequence, regardless of known function. Under the patent requirements that now stand, oligonucleotide sequences are patentable material. Theoretically, anyone could compose oligonucleotides of a distinct length, say 20 bases. Since oligonucleotides of that complexity would, in theory, occur only once in the human genome, each sequence could represent a unique segment of the genome and could possibly code for a segment of a disease gene. Using computers, every conceivable permutation of a 20-base sequence could be generated and patents requested. The granting of such patents may preclude the obtaining of oligonucleotide patents by researchers who have determined the oligonucleotide sequence that identifies a disease mutation. This seems illogical and contrary to the spirit with which patent rights were first conceived. But in essence this is what the patent application by NIH is attempting to do, except that the DNA sequences are several hundred base pairs in length, and they are known to be found in a gene. If an individual could only file a patent for a single DNA sequence at a time, such an attempt to monopolize future gene discoveries would be cost prohibitive. But the current patent laws do not protect scientists who have invested extensive labor efforts from exploitation by individuals not involved in the research.

Even if a middle ground could be found that would balance the protection awarded by the patent with the requirement for prior knowledge of the protein encoded by the gene, one could possibly circumvent the patent. Because of the redundancy of the genetic code, it is possible to extensively alter a DNA sequence for a gene without changing the amino acid composition of the protein. This must obviously be considered a new DNA sequence that could be patented. Such an action would nullify any patent royalties that might be gained by the first group.

This logic could be pursued even further. If one group of researchers filed a patent for a gene, could another group file a patent for the protein encoded by the gene, and yet another group file a patent on the experimental method used for the overexpression of that protein? Could another group reasonably be denied a patent for making the protein using a protein synthesizer because its product was obtained by a different approach? These are conceivable possibilities because science is an ongoing process characterized by continual advances, modifications, and extensions of previous research efforts. If patenting became the norm, where would it end? Clearly, definitive guidelines would have to be developed as to what material could be covered by the patent.

Will Patenting Inhibit Research?

It is important to remember that scientific research is not performed in a vacuum. New strategies may be designed and implemented, but almost all experiments are based on the work of others.

Medical research is different from other forms of research in that most of the work is performed in universities and institutions whose aim is to enhance the knowledge of who we are and what we are. Research functions by peer review and is energized by many informal discussions that take place daily and during scientific meetings. If this field becomes patent-happy, there is no question that barriers to the flow of information will occur. Even now, when requests are made for the sharing of biological samples, material transfer agreements are becoming more common. This protects the right of the individual who is sending the sample, but it occurs at the cost of delaying progress and preventing scientists from utilizing the entire scope of their creative talent. While material transfer agreements are not patents, the use of these agreements impose limitations that might be similar to patents.

Another delay caused by the patent process is that researchers may decide to file a patent application before they publish their research data. This in fact interposes patent lawyers between the discovery and the dissemination of the results. The real problem is that by withholding potentially important scientific discoveries, scientists delay the work of other scientists that might lead to additional insights about a disease. The dilemma of sharing information with other competitors occurs even without the issue of patent applications, but it is clear that science progresses at a much more rapid pace when competition is fostered and when the recognition goes to the scientist that reached the goal first.

If the DNA sequence for a common disease gene is identified and financial gain may result from the eventual marketing of a genetic test, scientists may delay publishing this information until a patent application can be filed. Although U.S. law grants a person the right to file for a patent up to one year after publication, some researchers may feel the need for immediate patent filing even though the U.S. law grants patents to the person first to invent rather than first to file. Is this potential delay for financial rewards acceptable in a field that is based on attempts to increase the quality of life?

If patenting becomes standard practice, it will be important to develop rules that protect the researcher's interest but do not impede scientific progress.

Who Should Obtain the Patent Rights?

In the area of medicine, where cooperation and collaboration are so essential, should a scientist who has "found" the code for a gene be allowed to gain exclusive rights to that gene and all the manipulations involving the gene? To understand this concern, it is important to know what is involved in identifying a specific disease gene. The following is a description of some of the steps needed to find a gene using positional cloning techniques, an approach used extensively in modern medical research:

1. First, individuals or families who have the disease must be identified, and the initial diagnosis confirmed. Following confirmation of the diagnosis, a biological sample must be obtained from each individual. This usually involves collecting and processing a blood sample so that a permanent cell line can be obtained. Recruiting patients to participate in such a research endeavor is not a trivial process; it demands the time of skilled clinicians for patient contacts and the collection of samples. The contribution of clinical staff to any research project cannot be overlooked.

2. Once the biological samples are available, the process of locating the disease gene begins. This process is technically demanding and requires skill and patience. It is necessary to screen many random DNA probes until one is found that is close enough to be coinherited with the disease gene. Sometimes one is lucky, as in the case with Huntington's disease where the eighth probe showed linkage with the disease. In most cases, however, years can be spent trying to find a reliable marker near the disease.

3. After a linked marker has been found, the next step is to proceed to locate the chromosomal region that harbors the disease gene. Again, years can be spent on further efforts to localize the defect. These efforts require the talents and time of technicians, graduate students, and postdoctoral researchers.

4. After defining the precise chromosomal region that contains the gene, it is necessary to identify which of the genes in the region is "the" disease gene. Proof usually requires the identification of the mutation that can explain why the gene is defective. These experiments involve rigorous analysis of affected and unaffected individuals to ensure that the mutation has in fact been identified.

Because the discovery of a medically significant gene depends on the collaboration and cooperation among a large number of individuals, identifying the rightful owner who may claim patentable rights to the gene is a daunting task. At present, the institutions with whom the lab director is affiliated are usually rewarded with patent rights. The institutions may share the patent rights with the lab director or additional key personnel. Such patent ownership is usually covered by employment agreements. However, no consideration is usually given to the long list of laboratories that have provided key information that leads to the discovery of the gene.

It is surprising, however, to note that the agencies that have financially backed the research endeavors are excluded from patent consideration. While they may retain the right to use the technology free from royalties, no financial gain is shared with these agencies. Such funding for research usually comes from NIH, nonprofit organizations, foundations that are financed by individual donations, and the universities that hire scientists and support their research efforts in indirect ways. If these agencies fund the research, should they not also have some share of the patent ownership and any royalties that might result from the patent?

Conclusions

From the point of view of a scientist in the field of human genetics, the most important aspect of our research is to provide the community with all the available information about a specific disease in a timely manner in order to offer diverse and affordable choices for treatment and testing. Expenses for medical treatment are skyrocketing, and the patenting of DNA sequences would only add to this problem. It may be best for the medical community and the community at large if no patenting were allowed for biological material. This is an extreme opinion and the consequences may not all be positive, but it may allow the free flow of information and let scientists pursue their goals unhindered by patent concerns. However, if no patents existed for biological material, biotechnology companies could exploit these discoveries for their own financial gains with no compensation for the individuals involved in research. This circumstance argues against the no-patent policy, but is this necessarily bad? Since both NIH and nonprofit organizations are funded by public monies through taxation or donations, the people should have the access to and use of this information without additional charges imposed by patents. It is also in the public interest to make information available to other scientists so that further advances can be made.

If there must be patents, then strict regulations must be implemented so that scientific progress is not delayed. There is no question that biotechnology companies that invest great sums of money in research and development expect to make a profit. But should there be a limit on the extent to which financial profits can be obtained from such research? It would not seem unreasonable to estimate the amount of money spent on the development of the company's product, be it a drug or a DNA sequence, and then to set limits on the profit that can be obtained from its commercial exploitation. Once the company reaches this limit, the patent would expire. It should be noted that companies perform research and development on many products that are never marketable, and it is the successful products that cover the costs of the unsuccessful products. Thus, it would be important to consider the entire research and development budget of the company. In the case of a university or institution, similar standards could apply for the ability to charge royalties based on the level of financial commitment made to the research endeavor. In this case, the patent would expire after the initial financial expenditures were completely recovered.

It does not seem unreasonable to suggest that the agencies that fund research should share in the financial gains of such efforts. One advantage of such a policy would be that the monies gained from royalties could then be reinvested in other research projects, thus increasing the level of research that can be supported by NIH, NSF (National Science Foundation), as well as other private, nonprofit organizations.

It is unfortunate that, despite their contributions toward exciting medical advances that hold promise of increasing the quality of life, scientists are faced with uncertainty about the impact of patents. Most scientists do not enter the field for the financial rewards of patent royalties. They pursue a career in science because they have a thirst for knowledge; their motivation reflects a desire to understand how the world functions. It is a grave concern that paranoia may creep into this exciting profession as scientists may need to look over their shoulders and ask whether some new finding is patentable. It is hard to imagine the free flow of ideas amidst suspicions of a collaborator or competitor who may be planning to apply for a patent using scientific information obtained by others.

12

Intellectual Property and Human Dignity

Ted Peters, Ph.D., M.Div.

Kate Murashige should be commended for striving diligently to maintain a dialectic between the individual trees and the whole forest, between the more limited patent policy considerations and considerations involving the encompassing global good. Specifically, she concludes that patent protection for intellectual property will (1) affect the amount of effort put into research; (2) impact the manner in which the economic system will structure itself; and (3) influence public and professional attitudes toward various ethical issues. Then, with these three trees in mind, she looks at the forest by forecasting a possible significant impact on the nature of society and even on global ecology. The threshold issue, she says, is this: To what extent is intellectual property protection for processes related to genetic testing and manipulation desirable?

The current controversy seems to have been sparked by the initial filing in June 1991 for patent property rights on 337 genes, and a second filing in February 1992 on 2,375 more genes by J. Craig Venter. Venter's research at NIH's National Institute of Neurological Disorders and Strokes aimed at locating and sequencing the 30,000 or so complementary DNAs, or cDNAs, from the human brain. These cDNAs are clones made from messenger RNAs; thus, they represent the coding regions of all the genes expressed in a tissue. By sequencing a short stretch of cDNA clones, about 300 to 500 bases, Venter has created what he calls an "expressed sequence tag," or EST. The automatic sequencing machine he uses churns out 50 to 150 tags per day, and this appears to be speeding up the task of locating the 100,000 or so estimated genes in the human genome. The patent application for protection of this new knowledge has generated a number of questions, some hotly debated. A preliminary U.S. Patent and Trademark Office ruling in the fall of 1992 denied the applications on the grounds that gene fragments cannot be patented without a known function. Since then Bernadine Healy, when still director of the National Institutes of Health, pressed for an appeal; and Incyte Pharmaceuticals Inc. of Palo Alto, California, began what might become a trend in the private sector of filing for patents on gene sequences. Two intertwined but distinguishable issues are these: Should patents be granted for knowledge of gene sequences at all? And, if so, should they be granted to a government-funded agency such as NIH or only to the private sector?

Hotly Debated Questions

First, does successful cDNA sequencing count as decisive knowledge about the genes themselves? Venter is the first to admit that, even though he can tag a cDNA, he still has no idea what it does, unless it is a sequence from a gene whose function is already known. James D. Watson, who opposes this rush to patent, decries the overvaluing of what has been accomplished (1992). Simply sequencing a short piece of an unidentified clone with an automated sequencing machine is a "dumb, repetitive task" (Roberts 1991, 184). What remains to be done and what remains decisive, he says, is to interpret the data so that we learn exactly what function each gene performs. Similarly, members of the Gene Patent Working Group, an interagency committee set up by the White House Office of Science and Technology Policy (OSTP), meeting in May 1992, said that ESTs are merely research tools and should not be granted patent protection that belongs to knowledge of the complete gene sequence and function (Zurer 1992, 21).(1) In short, critics argue, patenting at this stage is premature. Second, is this particular intellectual knowledge patentable? To patent, an invention must meet three criteria: it must be novel, nonobvious, and have utility. Certainly Venter's application is novel because the newly identified genes seem not to have been sequenced before. However, it is less obvious that it is nonobvious. Venter is making application of existing technology; he did not invent it. Nevertheless, Venter has contributed an insight that has led to unprecedented speed in scientific searching ability. This must be worth something, his sponsoring lawyers argue. Yet this does not speak to the toughest hurdle, utility. Venter's genes have been dubbed "naked," meaning that their function remains unknown. Until the function is known, no movement can be made toward developing medical or other benefits (Anderson 1991, 485).

Third, should intellectual knowledge regarding natural processes in principle be patentable? Does witnessing an existing natural phenomenon in itself warrant patent protection for the witness? Recalling that Sir Edmund Hillary and Tenzing Norgay were the first mountain climbers to see the top of Mount Everest on March 29, 1953, one might ask by analogy: Should Hillary and Norgay have been able to patent Mount Everest? Kate Murashige raises this issue by distinguishing between discovery and invention. The human genome is not invented; rather, it is in the process of being discovered by scientists. Like Mount Everest, it was already there. The discovery might be new, but the phenomenon of nature is itself not novel. Murashige reports that legal precedents seem to have been set in behalf of patenting the intellectual products of DNA discoveries. However, one might still pose the philosophical question: Should it be this way? Does this general principle apply to cDNAs? Perhaps cDNAs will be exempt. The cDNA is a copy version of the gene with the introns edited out. It does not occur naturally. It is coded into messenger RNA by the process that reads the raw cellular DNA. This leads Daniel Kevles and Leroy Hood (1992, 313) to argue: "Since it can be physically realized by a devising of human beings, using the enzyme reverse transcriptase, it is patentable." Yet Kevles and Hood are troubled:

> At first glance, the reasons might seem obvious: if anything is literally a common birthright of human beings, it is the human genome. It would thus seem that if anything should be avoided in the genomic political economy, it is a war of patents and commerce over the operational elements of that birthright (314).

In sum, cDNAs may prove to be patentable on the grounds that they are the product of a humanly devised process of gaining intellectual knowledge. As long as the principle holds that processes already occurring in nature are exempt, the human genome itself will not become patentable.

Fourth, should the U.S. National Institutes of Health encourage such patent applications? Former NIH Director Bernadine Healy says yes. Her policy is that NIH-funded researchers such as Venter should file for patents prior to publication. James Watson says no. Watson has blasted the initial filing as a land grab, a preemptive strike that will likely promote a worldwide stampede to garner patents on essentially meaningless pieces of DNA (1992). The basic problem is that this policy will foster secrecy among scientists; it will destroy the fragile practice of open sharing of information among scientists around the world (Roberts 1992, 912).(2)

Watson is not alone in his criticism. French geneticist Daniel Cohen speaks for many critics when he tells the press that there are two big problems with the NIH approach to patenting:

> The first is moral. You can't patent something that belongs to everyone. It's like trying to patent the stars. The second is economic. By patenting something without knowing the use of it, you inhibit industry. This could be a catastrophe (Thompson 1993, 57).

Even the National Institutes of Health Department of Energy Subcommittee for Interagency Coordination of the Human Genome

Initiative, meeting on January 3, 1992, declared:

> We are unanimous in deploring the decision to seek such patents. . . . Our immediate concern is that the filing of such claims undermines the activities of the Human Genome Project. There is also a strong likelihood that the pursuit of such patents will set off an international "patent race" and thereby compromise or destroy the international collaboration that we regard as essential for the work ahead (Roberts 1992, 913).

This is certainly not the way Healy sees it. The long-range goal of NIH is to encourage development of products for treating disease. In the short range though, Healy argues that, by applying for patents on Venter's work, NIH can release his data to other scientists while still preserving intellectual property rights. Reid Adler, director of the NIH Office of Technology Transfer, contends that there is no need for such an uproar. The NIH practice of patent filing is only an interim policy, he says, that is designed to protect its researchers until a permanent policy is adopted. That permanent policy may even reverse the current one, with the result that these patent applications would be dropped. In the meantime, NIH wishes to clarify two misconceptions. First, researchers are free to conduct studies on any gene they wish, even if patented. Second, Adler's reading of patent law is that partial sequences with tags are indeed patentable and could give rights to the entire gene (Veggeberg 1992, 9). The upshot seems to be that the policy is process, awaiting a legal decision. (3)

While we wait, international negotiators are charged with the task of bringing greater uniformity to the worldwide patenting process. The United Nations World Intellectual Property Organization (WIPO) along with the General Agreements on Tariffs and Trade (GATT) are tackling such issues as first to invent versus first to file. American patent law gives priority to the person who can prove with a notarized laboratory notebook or similar evidence that he or she made the invention first. Most other nations give priority to the one who first makes application for a patent. (4) While these and other matters are discussed, and uniform policy regarding property rights over DNA sequencing is at best a hope for the future, other nations are eyeing the United States with suspicion and considering defensive maneuvers. David Owen of the United Kingdom's Medical Research Council (MRC) says his government wants an international agreement that no country will seek patents on gene sequences of unknown utility. In the meantime, however, the British government will be filing patent applications to protect its own claims. It will drop such claims if and when an appropriate international agreement is reached (Zurer 1992, 22). This means, among other things, that both advocates and critics of the patenting idea want to see this controversy pressed through to the end, even to the U.S. Supreme Court if need be, so that a uniform policy will help keep open an unimpeded flow of scientific information.

Should We Alter God's Creatures?

Kate Murashige notes that "while human beings cannot be patented, techniques for manipulating them can." She thinks it is a bit odd that human beings cannot be patented. It is inconsistent with two principles, one scientific and one legal. The scientific principle is that a continuity and relatedness exists that binds all life together; all organisms, from the lowliest bacterium to the most elevated human, translate the same genetic code in the same way. The legal principle is that we quite unemotionally manipulate plant genes and we emotionally manipulate animal genes, patenting the results of both. Despite ethical objections raised by animal-rights advocates and others, the patenting of unicellular and now even multicellular creatures such as the Harvard mouse have set precedents for further patenting of invented life forms. (5) Yet this step has not been taken with regard to granting intellectual property rights over a human being. Perhaps one could pose the issue this way: either one should be able to patent all invented living creatures, humans included, or none.

Murashige suggests that those who see "sinister implications in genetic manipulation of living creatures" such as plants and animals may have the better insight. When they argue against "interference with divine creation," they seem to be acknowledging the continuity and relatedness of all living things, human beings included.

Although this is a tributary aside from the central flow of the Murashige chapter, the concept of "interference with divine creation" warrants some exploration. Those most concerned with the concept of divine creation and our responsibility toward it are theologians and ethicists in the churches and other religious communities. What have they said with regard to inventing new, useful, and nonobvious human beings?

Relevant here is the debate regarding the relationship between somatic therapy and germline enhancement. "Somatic therapy" refers to the treatment of a disease in the body cells of a living individual by trying to repair an existing defect. "Germline enhancement" refers to intervention into the germline cells that would influence heredity and improve the quality of life for future generations.

Numerous ethical interpreters agree that somatic therapy is morally desirable, and they look forward to the advances gene research will bring for expanding this important medical work. Yet many who reflect on the ethical implications of the new genetic research stop short of endorsing genetic selection and manipulation for the purposes of improving the human species. Molecular hematologist W. French Anderson speaks for many when he says (1990, 23):

> Somatic cell gene therapy for the treatment of severe disease is considered ethical because it can be supported by the fundamental moral principle of beneficence: It would relieve human suffering. Gene therapy would be,

therefore, a moral good. Under what circumstances would human genetic engineering not be a moral good? In the broadest sense, when it detracts from, rather than contributes to, the dignity of man. . . . Somatic cell enhancement engineering would threaten important human values in two ways: It could be medically hazardous. . . . And it would be morally precarious, in that it would require moral decisions our society is not now prepared to make, and it could lead to an increase in inequality and discriminatory practices.

In short, genetic enhancement risks violating human dignity by opening up the possibility of discrimination.

The concept of dignity is decisive here. With regard to "dignity" one thinks of the Enlightenment principle that a human being is to be treated as an end, not a means to a further end. The modern humanist understanding of dignity is in part a secularization of the previous religious commitment to the infinite value of the human soul. What this means is that a human person is the locus and end of moral value, not to be subordinated to other values presumed to be higher. Murashige does not refer to dignity in her discussion, but one can presume that the present proscription against patenting human beings derives from human dignity. In modern Western culture, it is primarily dignity, not genes, that separates the human being from plants and animals.

Theological ethicists who have addressed the issue similarly argue that somatic therapy should be pursued, but enhancement through germline engineering raises cautions. Although the appeal to human dignity is implicit, it alone does not drive the argument against germline intervention. The World Council of Churches (WCC) is representative as displayed in the following 1982 document (6-7):

Somatic cell therapy may provide a good; however, other issues are raised if it also brings about a change in germ-line cells. The introduction of genes into the germ-line is a permanent alteration. . . . Nonetheless, changes in genes that avoid the occurrence of disease are not necessarily made illicit merely because those changes also alter the genetic inheritance of future generations. . . . There is no absolute distinction between eliminating "defects" and "improving" heredity. (6)

Elsewhere in the text, the WCC is primarily concerned with humanity's lack of knowledge regarding the possible consequences of altering the human germline. The problem is this: the present generation lacks sufficient information regarding the long-term consequences of a decision today that might turn out to be irreversible tomorrow. Thus, the WCC does not forbid germline therapy or even enhancement forever. Rather, it cautions us to wait and see. In similar fashion, the Methodists "support human gene therapies that produce changes that cannot be passed on to offspring (somatic), but believe that they should be limited to the alleviation of suffering caused by disease" (United Methodist 1992, 121). The United Church of Christ also approves "altering cells in the human body, if the alteration is not passed to offspring" (1989, 3). (7)

The Catholic Health Association is more positive: If human health can be improved through germline intervention, then it is morally desirable:

> Germ-line intervention is potentially the only means of treating genetic diseases that do their damage early in embryonic development, for which somatic cell therapy would be ineffective. Although still a long way off, developments in molecular genetics suggest that this is a goal toward which biomedicine could reasonably devote its efforts (Catholic Health Association 1990, 19).

The history of eugenics also makes religiously sensitive people cautious about germline enhancement. The term "eugenics" brings to mind the ghastly racial policies of Nazism, and this accounts for much of today's mistrust of genetic science in Germany and elsewhere (Kevles 1992; Meyer 1991). No one expects a repeat of Nazi terror to emerge from genetic engineering; yet some critics fear a subtle form of eugenics may be slipping in the cultural backdoor (Duster 1990; Rifkin 1983). The growing power to control the human genetic make-up could foster the emergence of the image of the "perfect child" or a "super strain" of humanity; and the impact of the social value of perfection will begin to oppress all those who fall short. Ethicists at the March 1992 conference on "Genetics, Religion and Ethics" held at the Texas Medical Center in Houston said this:

> Because the Jewish and Christian religious world-view is grounded in the equality and dignity of individual persons, genetic diversity is respected. Any move to eliminate or reduce human diversity in the interest of eugenics or creating a "super strain" of human being will meet with resistance.

In sum, religious ethicists reflecting on germline enhancement over the last decade are committed to maintaining human dignity, and this seems to extend to the point of saying no to intervention into the genetic make-up of future generations even if that intervention improves human health and well-being. With the possible exception of the Catholic Health Association, religious ethical thinking tends to be conservative in the sense that it seeks to conserve the present pool of genes on the human genome for the indefinite future.

What are the implications of this ethical discussion for the future of patents? If this viewpoint holds sway, it will discourage the attempt to invent a better human being through genetic manipulation and thereby discourage its accompanying patent practice. Even apart from discouraging such dramatic interventions such as eugenic enhancement through germline alteration, the concept of human dignity will continue to severely limit the scope of intellectual property rights over the human genome, at least when compared to rights over plants or animals. Will this conservative religious viewpoint continue to dominate? Not necessarily, although forecasting the future on such a matter is difficult. Relevant to

this discussion is an emerging alternative theological view that empha-
sizes the continuing character of God's creative activity—the doctrine of
creatio continua—plus the cooperative role that the human race plays in
this divine creative activity. If God can be understood as the world's
creator, and if the human race can be understood as created in God's
image, then creative activity befits the ongoing human contribution to
this world. With this in mind, theologian Philip Hefner (1989) has begun
naming the human being the "created co-creator."(8) Not only is the
present generation of human beings the product of a long history of
evolution, in the future, society will at least in part share the responsibility
of what we as a race will become. The creative process continues. We have
the capacity, among other things, of altering the genetic make-up of
future generations. Should we do it? Does this theological understanding
of ongoing creation imply an ethic of deliberate self-creativity? If the
answer becomes yes, and if this viewpoint begins to hold sway in religious
communities, one might find a rethinking of the proscription against
germline enhancement. There might be new pressure to ponder again the
propriety of inventing and patenting new human beings.(9) If thumbs go
up, then one might add distinctively religious motives to pursuing genome
research on behalf of the betterment of the human race.

A further observation is added: The doctrine of human dignity may
not remain the private possession of the conservatives. If dignity means
that the human person is treated as an end rather than a means, then
arguments against enhancement based on such things as genetic diversity will fail. Once better health or well-being is envisioned and processes
of genetic alteration can be demonstrated to attain better health or well-
being, then how could it be denied on ethical grounds? The concept of
dignity may itself provide the ethical warrant for the creative engineering
of future generations.

Conclusion

Kate Murashige's threshold issue, recall, is this: to what extent is
intellectual property protection regarding gene research desirable? On
the basis of what has been said thus far, one can conclude with the
following thesis: insofar as patent protection encourages the worldwide
flow of information that enhances research everywhere—especially research aimed at improving human health and well-being—it is desirable;
insofar as it blocks or impedes that information-sharing, it is undesirable.

Notes

1. One critic, Jonathan Marc Rothberg, notes that Venter, perhaps unknow-
   ingly, appears to be applying for patents on at least eight Bluescript
   sequencing vectors already owned by Stratagene (Rothberg 1992, 738).

2. James Watson has sought all along to maximize information-sharing on a worldwide basis. He writes, "As soon as a gene has been identified, it should be thrown into an international data base" (Kevles and Hood 1992, 172). With this commitment, one can easily understand why Watson perceives a possible patent war as a significant obstacle.

3. In an interesting turn of events, Craig Venter resigned as section chief and laboratory chief at NIH's National Institute of Neurological Disorders and Strokes to take a position in private industry. He took over as head of The Institute for Genomic Research (TIGR), in Montgomery County, Maryland. In a statement released July 6, 1992, Bernadine Healy said, "The innovative technology pioneered by Dr. Craig Venter in NIH's intramural laboratories has truly come of age. Now it is time for Dr. Venter to take his bold discoveries out of NIH, a great marketplace of ideas, and into the marketplace of America, private industry." Venter told reporters he is leaning toward patent sequenced fragments in the future and that "the goal of the institute is not to try to monopolize or own human genes" (Hamilton 1992, 151).

4. Patents need not impede the flow of scientific information. In the event the United States should adopt the first-to-file policy, as Murashige suggests, it could include the requirement that, at the moment of filing, each patent would go into a common database and become available immediately to the worldwide scientific community. The problem is not the patent per se but rather the abuse of exclusivity that can accompany it. A statutory exemption for research purposes may be sufficient to blunt the tendency toward secrecy.

5. In December 1992, the U.S. Patent and Trademark Office broke a moratorium on patenting animals and issued patents to three organizations covering "transgenic" mice specially suited to medical research.

6. A 1989 document reiterates this position more strongly by proposing "a ban on experiments involving genetic engineering of the human germline at the present time" (World Council of Churches 1989, 2).

7. See also the interpretation and commentary on this pronouncement by Ronald Cole-Turner (1991). He also tracks some of the controversy over germline intervention (Cole-Turner 1993).

8. Hefner by no means conflates God and humanity. God creates *ex nihilo*, from nothing. We humans only transform what already exists. Both enterprises deserve the word "creation."

9. The doctrine of human dignity will not permit exclusive patent rights over an individual, of course. A modified genome formula is referred to here that would be shared by large numbers of people whose individual rights would remain intact.

References

Anderson, C. 1991. "To Patent a Naked Gene." *Nature* 353:485.

Anderson, W.F. 1990. "Genetics and Human Malleability." *Hastings Center Report* 20:21–24.

Catholic Health Association. 1990. *Human Genetics: Ethical Issues in Genetic Testing, Counseling, and Therapy.* St. Louis, MO: The Catholic Health Association of the United States.

Cole-Turner, R. 1993. *The New Genesis: Theology and the Genetic Revolution.* Louisville, KY: Westminster/John Knox Press.

Cole-Turner, R. 1991. "Genetics and the Church." *Prism* 6:53–61.

Duster, T. 1990. *Backdoor to Eugenics.* New York and London: Routledge.

Hamilton, D., ed. 1992. "Venter to Leave NIH for Greener Pastures." *Science* 257:151.

Hefner, P. 1989. "The Evolution of the Created Co-Creator." In T. Peters, ed., *Cosmos as Creation: Theology and Science in Consonance,* 211–234. Nashville, TN: Abingdon.

Institute of Religion and Baylor College of Medicine. 1992. "Summary Reflection Statement." Genetics, Religion, and Ethics Project. The Texas Medical Center, P.O. Box 20569, Houston, Texas 77225.

Kelves, D.J. 1992. "Out of Eugenics: The Historical Politics of the Human Genome." In D.J. Kelves and L. Hood, eds., *The Code of Codes: Scientific and Social Issues in the Human Genome Project.* Cambridge: Harvard University Press.

Kevles, D.J. and Hood, L., eds. 1992. *The Code of Codes: Scientific and Social Issues in the Human Genome Project.* Cambridge: Harvard University Press.

Meyer, P. 1991. "Biotechnology: History Shapes German Opinion." *Forum for Applied Research and Public Policy* (Winter) 6:92–97.

Rifkin, J. 1983. *Algeny.* New York: Viking.

Roberts, L. 1992. "NIH Gene Patents, Round Two." *Science* 255:912.

Roberts, L. 1991. "Genome Patent Fight Erupts." *Science* 254:184–186.

Rothberg, J.M. 1992. Letter. "Gene Patents." *Nature* 356:738.

Thompson, R. 1993. "The Race to Map Our Genes." *Time* 141:57.

United Church of Christ. 1989. "The Church and Genetic Engineering." Pronouncement of the Seventeenth General Synod, United Church of Christ, Fort Worth, Texas.

United Methodist Church. 1992. "United Methodist Church Genetic Task Force Report to the 1992 General Conference."

Veggeberg, S. 1992. "Controversy Mounts Over Gene Patenting Policy." *The Scientist* 6:9.

Watson, J. 1992. "A Personal View of the Project." In D.J. Kelves and L. Hood, eds., *The Code of Codes: Scientific and Social Issues in the Human Genome Project.* Cambridge: Harvard University Press.

World Council of Churches. 1989. "Biotechnology: Its Challenges to the Churches and the World."

World Council of Churches. 1982. *Manipulating Life: Ethical Issues in Genetic Engineering.* Geneva: WCC.

Zurer, P. 1992. "Critics Take Aim at NIH's Gene Patenting Strategy." *Chemical & Engineering News* 70:21–22.

Appendix

Individuals Associated with the AAAS—ABA Conference on Frontier Issues in Ethics, Law, and Genetic Testing

V. Elving Anderson[1]
Professor Emeritus
Department of Genetics and
Cell Biology
University of Minnesota
Minneapolis, Minnesota

R. Stephen Berry[4]
Professor
Department of Chemistry
University of Chicago
Chicago, Illinois

Alan Beyerchen[3]
Professor
History Department
Ohio State University
Columbus, Ohio

Joseph L. Birman[3]
Professor
Department of Physics
City College—City University of
New York
New York, New York

John H. Bodley[3]
Professor
Department of Anthropology
Washington State University
Pullman, Washington

Jane Bortnick Griffith[3]
Assistant Chief
Science Policy Research Division
Congressional Research Service
Library of Congress
Washington, DC

Elizabeth Gehman[1]
Executive Assistant to the Director
Directorate for Science & Policy
Programs
American Association for the
Advancement of Science
Washington, DC

The Honorable Ruth C. Burg[5]
Administrative Law Judge
Armed Services Board of
Contract Appeals
Falls Church, Virginia

Nina Byers[3]
Professor
Department of Physics
University of California
Los Angeles, California

Audrey Chapman[1]
Program Director
Science & Human Rights
Directorate for Science & Policy
Programs
American Association for the
Advancement of Science
Washington, DC

R. Alta Charo[1]
Professor of Law and Medical Ethics
University of Wisconsin
Madison, Wisconsin

Richard P. Claude[3]
Professor Emeritus
University of Maryland
College Park, MD

Ronald S. Cole-Turner[1]
Associate Professor of Theology
Memphis Theological Seminary
Memphis, Tennessee

Robert Cook-Deegan[1,2]
Director
Division of Biobehavioral Sciences
& Mental Disorders
Institute of Medicine
Washington, DC

Larry L. Deaven[1]
Deputy Director
Center for Human Genome Studies
Los Alamos National Laboratory
Los Alamos, New Mexico

Clarence J. Dias[3]
President
International Center for Law in
Development
New York, New York

Troy Duster[1]
Director
Institute for the Study of Social
Change
University of California
Berkeley, California

Andrea Bear Field[5]
Attorney
Hunton & Williams
Washington, DC

Ellen J. Flannery[5]
Attorney
Covington & Burling
Washington, DC

Alexander R. Fowler[1]
Program Assistant
Scientific Freedom, Responsibility
& Law
Directorate for Science & Policy
Programs
American Association for the
Advancement of Science
Washington, DC

Mark S. Frankel[1]
Program Director
Scientific Freedom, Responsibility
& Law
Directorate for Science & Policy
Programs
American Association for the
Advancement of Science
Washington, DC

Bernard Gert[1]
*Stone Professor of Intellectual and Moral
Philosophy*
Department of Philosophy
Dartmouth College
Hannover, New Hampshire

Ruth Greenstein[1,2,4]
*Vice President for Administration
& Finance*
Institute for Defense Analyses
Alexandria, Virginia

C.K. (Tina) Gunsalus[3]
Associate Vice Chancellor for Research
University of Illinois
Champaign, Illinois

Neil A. Holtzman[1,2]
Professor
Johns Hopkins Medical Institutions
Baltimore, Maryland

Arthur Horwich[2]
Associate Professor
Department of Human Genetics
School of Medicine
Yale University
New Haven, Connecticut

Sheila Jasanoff[1,2]
Chair
Department of Science &
Technology Studies
Cornell University
Ithaca, New York

Robert H. Kirschner[3]
Cook County Medical Examiner
Office
Chicago, Illinois

John Ladd[3]
Professor Emeritus
Department of Philosophy
Brown University
Providence, Rhode Island

Alan I. Leshner[1,4]
Deputy Director
National Institute of Mental Health
Rockville, Maryland

Sue Levi-Pearl[1]
Liaison, Medical & Scientific Programs
Tourette Syndrome Association
Bayside, New York

Abby Lippman[1]
Professor
Department of Epidemiology
and Biostatistics
McGill University
Montreal, Quebec
Canada

Lee Loevinger[1,5]
Attorney
Hogan & Hartson
Washington, DC

Harold Lurie[4]
Associate Director
California Council on Science
& Technology
Irvine, California

Richard A. Meserve[1,4]
Attorney
Covington & Burling
Washington, DC

William W. Middleton[3]
Consulting Engineer
St. Davids, Pennsylvania

Norval Morris[1]
*Julius Kreeger Professor of Law
and Criminology*
University of Chicago Law School
Chicago, Illinois

Kate Murashige[1]
Attorney
Morrison & Foerster
Washington, DC

Thomas H. Murray[1,2]
Director
Center for Biomedical Ethics
Case Western Reserve University
School of Medicine
Cleveland, Ohio

Susan H. Nycum[5]
Attorney
Baker & McKenzie
Palo Alto, California

Gilbert S. Omenn[1,2,4]
Dean
School of Public Health &
Community Medicine
University of Washington
Seattle, Washington

Pilar N. Ossorio[1]
Post Doctoral Associate
Division of Infectious Disease
Yale University School of Medicine
New Haven, Connecticut

Joan Overhauser[1]
Assistant Professor
Department of Biochemistry
& Molecular Biology
Thomas Jefferson University
Philadelphia, Pennsylvania

Ted Peters[1]
Professor of Systematic Theology
Pacific Lutheran Seminary
Berkeley, California

Madison Powers[1]
Senior Research Scholar
Kennedy Institute of Ethics
Georgetown University
Washington, DC

Denis J. Prager[4]
Director
Health Programs
John D. & Catherine T. MacArthur
Foundation
Chicago, Illinois

Stirling Puck[1]
Director of Cytogenetics
Vivigen, Inc.
Santa Fe, New Mexico

Kimberly A. Quaid[1,2]
*Clinical Assistant Professor of
Medical and Molecular Genetics
and Psychiatry*
Department of Medical Genetics
Indiana University School of
Medicine
Indianapolis, Indiana

John Robertson[1]
Thomas Watt Gregory Professor of Law
School of Law
University of Texas
Austin, Texas

Deborah Runkle[1]
Senior Program Associate
Scientific Freedom, Responsibility
& Law
Directorate for Science & Policy
Programs
American Association for the
Advancement of Science
Washington, DC

Charles A. Sanders[3]
Chairman & Chief Executive Officer
Glaxo, Inc.
Research Triangle Park, North
Carolina

Roger Shinn[1]
*Reinhold Niebuhr Professor of Social
Ethics Emeritus*
Union Theological Seminary
New York, New York

John F. Shoch[4]
General Partner
Asset Management Company
Palo Alto, California

Oliver R. Smoot[5]
Executive Vice President
Computer & Business Equipment
Manufacturers Association
Washington, DC

Laurence R. Tancredi[1,2]
Professor of Clinical Psychiatry
New York University Medical School
New York, New York

Albert H. Teich[1]
Director
Directorate for Science &
Policy Programs
American Association for the
Advancement of Science
Washington, DC

230

LeRoy Walters[2]
Director
Center for Bioethics
Kennedy Institute of Ethics
Georgetown University
Washington, DC

Robert A. Weinberg[2]
Professor of Biology
Whitehead Institute for
Biomedical Research
Massachusetts Institute of Technology
Cambridge, Massachusetts

Alan F. Westin[1]
Professor of Public Law and Government
Department of Political Science
Columbia University
New York, New York

Caroline Whitbeck[3]
Senior Lecturer
Mechanical Engineering
Massachusetts Institute of
Technology
Cambridge, Massachusetts

Thomas White[1]
Vice President of Research & Development
Roche Molecular Systems, Inc.
Alameda, California

Michael Yesley[1]
Coordinator, Ethical, Legal & Social Implications Program
Los Alamos National Laboratory
Los Alamos, New Mexico

Carl York[1]
Treasurer
Center for Theology and
the Natural Sciences
Berkeley, California

Nicholas C. Yost[5]
Dickstein, Shapiro & Morin
Washington, DC

Franklin M. Zweig[1]
Senior Fellow
Center for Health Policy Studies
George Washington University
Washington, DC

1. Participant in the American Association for the Advancement of Science/ American Bar Association Conference on Frontier Issues in Ethics, Law, and Genetic Testing
2. Advisory Committee to the Project on the Ethical and Legal Implications of Genetic Testing
3. Member of the American Association for the Advancement of Science Committee on Scientific Freedom and Responsibility, 1992
4. AAAS Member of the American Association for the Advancement of Science/American Bar Association National Conference of Lawyers and Scientists, 1992
5. ABA Member of the American Association for the Advancement of Science/American Bar Association National Conference of Lawyers and Scientists, 1992

Index

Academic genetic databanks, 88
Acquired immunodeficiency syndrome
        (AIDS), 11, 13-14, 17
Adler, Reid, 218
Adoption, 27, 29-30
    Vermont's adoption law, 40
African Americans
    anthropological view of blacks, 134
    incarceration rates of, 147
Agriculture infrastructure, 191
Alcoholism, 118-119
Alexander, Richard, 161
American Association for the
        Advancement of Science (AAAS),
        Genetic Testing Project, xiv-xv
American Bar Association, xv
American Breeder's Association, 144-145
Anderson, W. French, 219-220
Animal patents, 190
Anonymity, 56
    pedigree studies and the protection of,
        89-92
Anthropology, 133, 134
Antisocial personality disorder, 121
Arranged marriages, practice of, 13
Artificial insemination, 10
    by donor (AID), 13, 14, 32, 35, 37
Ashkenazi Jews, 12
Asians, alcoholism effects on, 118
"Assortative mating," 13
Augustine, 166
Australia, contract gestation case, 36
Autonomy, patient, 49-50
Autonomy interests, 83
Autosomal dominant conditions, 49

Baby M case, 32-33, 38
Barefoot case, 156

Barth, Karl, 167
Behavior
    alcoholism, 118-119
    criminality, 121-123
    fragile X syndrome, 115-116
    genes and, 105-107, 113-115
    genetic and environmental influences
        on, 103-104
    Huntington's disease, 116-117
    intelligence, 119-121
    schizophrenia, 117-118
    substance abuse, 117
Behavior genetics, 161-165, 169, 170
Binet tests, 121, 139
Biological Darwinism to social Darwinism,
        132-133
Biology of Moral Systems, The (Alexander), 161
Biotechnology and genetic engineering
        patents, 190-192
Blacks. *See* African Americans
Blame and punishment, 158
Bloom, Floyd, 107
Bodmer, Walter, 200
Bottom-up strategies, 124
Brain
    development of the, 106, 107-108
    genes and the, 107
    implications of neurogenetic
        research, 112
    neurogenetics, 111-112
    neuronal signaling, 108-110
    reductionism and responsibility,
        123-124
    studies of the cerebellum, 110-111

California
    egg donation programs in, 33
    involuntary sterilization programs in, 145

California Supreme Court on the
traditional family unit, 34
Calvert, Crispina, 33-34, 35, 37
Canalization, concept of, 115
Carol C., 36, 37
Carter, Jimmy, 16
Case Western Reserve University, 15
Catholic Health Association, 221
Cause, as term, 170
Certificate of Confidentiality, 86, 89
Cetus Corporation, 202
Chakrabarty oil-eating bacterium, 190
Chargaff, Erwin, 16
Children
and monogamy, 10
XYY, 122
Christianity, 135, 167
Churchland, Patricia, 124
Church, the
and human genetics, 134-135
theological ethicists on germline
enhancement, 220-221
Cloninger, Robert, 123
Cohen-Boyer patent, 185, 196, 202
Cohen, Daniel, 217
Cold Spring Harbor Laboratories, 200
Cole, R. David, 124
Collaborative Perinatal Project, 121
Collective rights, 94
Colon cancer, 47
Columbia University, 16, 18
Commission for the Study of Ethical
Problems in Medicine and
Biomedical and Behavioral
Research, 16
Composition-of-matter patents, 205
Confidentiality, 17, 49
"Continuation-in-part" patent application,
199-200
Contract motherhood, 32, 35
Moschetta case, 36-37
Copyright protection, 183
Creatio continua, doctrine of, 222
Criminal behavior, 155, 156-157
Criminality, 121-123
Criminal justice system, DNA testing
and the, 160

Criminal prosecution, 97
Cystic fibrosis (CF), 12, 47, 164, 165, 210
carrier screening for, 94

Darwin, Charles, 132-133, 167
Data protection codes, 60-61
Data protection commissions, European
system of, 63-64, 89
Davenport, Charles, 137-138
Defining the family after the genetic
revolution, 25-44
Delbanco, Andrew, 18
Depression, 11
Descartes, Rene, 167-168
Determinism
genetics and, 169-170
and responsibility, 171-172
Dignity, concept of, 220
Disclosure and surveillance, 57-58
Disclosures
collection and disclosure of genetic
information, 47-51
control over, 87-88
disclosure issues in research contexts,
88-90
information disclosed for the
protection of others, 92-93
Discrimination suits, 97
Disease genes, 209, 212
DNA databanks, 47, 87-88, 96, 97
DNA fingerprinting, 17, 47, 202
DNA, isolated and purified, 188
DNA sequences, 186, 187
NIH cDNA patent applications,
192-194, 199, 200, 215-216,
217-218
patents for, 209-214
DNA techniques, recombinant, 201-202
DNA testing and the criminal justice
system, 160
Dobzhansky, Theodosius, 125
Dopamine receptors, 109-110
alcoholism and, 118
Drosophila gene, 109
Dupont v. Cetus, 186
Durkheim, Emile, 135
Duster, Troy, 105

Edinburgh, Scotland, 146
Egg donation programs, 33, 35, 37
English common law, 29, 31
Environment on genes and behavior,
    106-107
Enzymes
    patented, 203
    restriction, 202
Ethical, Legal, and Social Issues (ELSI)
    program, xiv, 68
Ethics, subject of, 18-20
Eugenics, 14, 133, 221
European Community, Working Group
    of the, 4
European Data Protection Commission,
    63-64, 89
European immigration, 138-140, 145
European Patent Office, 183
Excitatory synaptic action, 109
"Expressed sequence tag" (EST), 215, 216
Eysenck, H. J., 142

Fair Credit Reporting Act of 1970, 63
Fair information practices, 60-61
Family
    biological model of the, 28
    biological relationships, discarding,
        30-32
    contractual model of the, 28-20
    genes and families, 3-7
    genetic model of the, 26-28
    and public policy needs, 37-39
Family relationships and social policy, 9-23
Farming and agriculture, 191
Federal Bureau of Investigation (FBI), 47
Federal Privacy Act of 1974, 61
First-to-invent/first-inventor-to-file
    systems, 195
Fisher, Ronald, 138
Food and Drug Administration
    (FDA), 190
Foster parents, 28
    Moschetta case, 36-37
Foundation of the Metaphysics of Morals
    (Kant), 168
Fragile X syndrome, 115-116
Franklin, Benjamin, 177
Frazer, James George, 134, 135

Freedom of Information Act, 62
French Declaration of Rights, 125

Galton, Francis, 133, 136, 137, 162,
    166-167
Gamma-aminobutyric acid (GABA),
    109, 119
Gay couples as parents, 11, 39-40
GenBank, 205
Gene mapping, 47, 113, 117-118
Gene patenting. *See* Patent protection in
    the United States
Gene Patent Working Group, White
    House Office of Science and
    Technology Policy (OSTP), 216
General Agreement on Tariffs and Trade
    (GATT), 183, 218
Genes
    behavior, and responsibility, 105-130
    Drosphila, 109
    and family, 3-7
    "immediate early," 106
    K-*ras* oncogene, 200
    mcf transforming, 200
    tagged, 107
Genes, Mind, and Culture
    (Wilson and Lumsden), 142
Genetical Theory of Natural Selection, The
    (Fisher), 138
Genetic determinism, 169-170
Genetic explanations, appropriation of,
    142-144
Genetic fingerprinting, 17, 47, 202
Genetic information
    collection and disclosure of, 47-51
    privacy and, 53-76
    privacy and the control of, 77-100
Genetic registries, 85-86
    nonresearch registries and databanks,
        89-90
Genetics
    behavior, and responsibility, 155-160
    crime, violence, and race, 146-148
    and determinism, 169-170
Genetics of moral agency, 161-174
Genetic specialization, areas of, 143-144
"Genetics, Religion and Ethics"
    conference, 221

Genetic testing and the Human Genome
    Project, xiii-xix
  of parents or prospective parents, 12-14
Genetic testing and intellectual property,
    181-198
  a commentary, 199-208
  a scientist's perspective, 209-214
Genetic therapy, 15-16
Genomic Research Institute, The (TIGR),
    193-194
Germany
  eugenics, 221
  eugenic sterilization law, 145-146
  misuse of genetic information about
  Huntington's disease in Nazi, 116
Germline cells, 16
"Germline enhancement," 219-221
Gestational surrogacy case, 33-34, 35
Gestational surrogacy programs, 35
"Gestation-vs.-genetics" debate, 37-38
Gladden, Washington, 166
Golden Bough, The (Frazer), 134, 135
Goodwin, Frederick, 11
Gordon, Robert, 142
Gottesman, Irving, 114, 115, 123
Gould, Stephen, 135-136

Harvard Law Review, 58
Harvard mouse patent, 190
Health care industry and the patent
    system, 196
Health insurance, reforms for, 96
Healy, Bernadine, 216, 217, 218
Hefner, Philip, 222
Heisenberg, Werner, 19
Hereditary Genius (Galton), 166-167
Herrnstein, Richard, 142
Hillary, Edmund, 216-217
Hoffman-LaRoche, 186
Holmes, Oliver Wendell, 133
Holmes, S. J., 145
Hood, Leroy, 217
Human dignity, intellectual property and,
    215-224
Human Genetic Diversity Project, 149
Human genetics, evolutionary theory, and
    social stratification, 131-153

Human Genome Project
  genetic testing and the, xiii-xix
  privacy analysis of the, 66-68
Human Genome Sciences, 193-194
Human germ cells, 16
Human population genetics and human
    Mendelian genetics, 136-142
Hume, David, 164, 168, 169
Huntington's disease (HD), 47, 84, 92,
    94-95, 116-117
Huntington's Disease Research Roster, 87
Huxley, Julian, 163

"Immediate early" genes, 106
Immigration, European, 138-140, 145
Incyte Pharmaceuticals, Inc., 216
Indiana University DNA Databank, 87
Individual privacy, four basic states of,
    56-57
Information disclosed for the protection
    of others, 92-93
Inhibitory synaptic action, 109
In re Chakrabarty, 190
In re Durden, 188-189
In re Pleuddemann, 189
In re Wiggins, 205, 206
Institutional Review Boards, 89, 90
Insurability, loss of, 96
Intellectual property and genetic testing,
    181-198
  a commentary, 199-208
  a scientist's perspective, 209-214
Intellectual property and human dignity,
    215-224
Intelligence, 119-121
"Interference" action, 201
International Committee of Medical
    Journal Editors, 90
Intimacy, 56
In vitro fertilization, 10-11, 15
IQ tests, 119-121, 139
Isolated and purified DNA, patents for, 188
Israel, genetic definition of motherhood, 38

Japanese Patent Office, 183
"Jeffreys" patent, 202
Jensen, Arthur, 134, 142

Johnson, Anna, 33-34, 35, 38, 39
Jordan, David Starr, 145
Jordan, Elvira, 36
Judaism, 27
Jurisdiction, problems of, 97

Kant, I., 168-169
Karp, J. P., 203
Kety, Seymour, 142
Kevles, Daniel, 217
Kiley, T. D., 204
Kinases, 111-112
"Knock-out" mice, 111-112
K-*ras* oncogene, 200

Lamarckian genetics, 162-163, 167
Lawsuits, 97
Lesbian couples as parents, 11, 40
Liberty rights, 83, 94, 95
Ligase chain reaction (LCR), pending
          patents for, 203
Linda K., 36
Linking genetics, behavior, and
          responsibility: legal implications,
          155-160
Locke, John, 167-168
Long-sleep (LS) lines, 118-119
Long-term potentiation (LTP), 111, 112
Louis Harris/Westin public opinion
          surveys on privacy, 62
Lucas, Malcolm M., 34
Lumsden, C. J., 142
Lysenko, T. D., 163

MacIntyre, A., 168
Mandatory minimum sentences, 157
Manipulation
     academia in genetic, 192-194
     genetic testing and, 185-187
     mcf transforming genes, 200
Mead, Margaret, 10
Mednick, Sarnoff, 142
Men
     alcoholism in, 118
     families headed by, 11
     and monogamy, 10
     XYY males, 146-147, 156-157

Mendel, Gregor, 136
Mendelian genetics, 136, 137, 138, 163
Mental illness and mental retardation, 156
Messenger RNA (mRNA), 107, 215, 217
Methodists on human gene therapies, 220
Method-of-use/method-to-make claims, 189
Milunsky, Aubrey, 146-147
Mismeasure of Man, The (Gould), 135-136
Molecular genetics, 110, 124, 142-144
Monogamy, 9-10
Moon, Sun Myung, 13
Moral agency, the genetics of, 161-174
Moral phenotype, 169, 170
Mormon polygamy, 10
Moschetta, Cynthia and Robert, 36
Motherhood, genetic definition of, 38-39
Mount Everest, 216-217
Muller, Herman, 14-16
Multiple parents, 39-41
Murashige, Kate, 181-198, 215, 219, 220

National Academy of Sciences, 144
National Conference of Lawyers and
          Scientists (NCLS), xv
National Council of the Churches of
          Christ in the U.S.A., 16
National Institute of Mental Health
          (NIMH), 11
     Research on Perpetrators of Violence
          program, 148
National Institutes of Health (NIH), xiv, 68
     cDNA patent applications, 192-194,
          199, 200, 215-216, 217-218
     Department of Energy Subcommittee for
          Interagency Coordination of the
          Human Genome Initiative
          meeting, 217-218
     and gene therapy, 16
     "Genetic Factors in Crime: Findings, Uses,
          and Implications" conference, 122
National Institute of Neurological
          Disorders and Strokes, 215
National Research and Education Network
          (NREN), 63
National Research Council (NRC), 122-123
National Science Foundation (NSF), 214
Natural parent, definition of, 35-37

"New," use of the term, 184
New Jersey Supreme Court, Mary Beth
    Whitehead case and the, 32
New York State Bar Association House of
    Delegates, 34
Niebuhr, Reinhold, 167
Nixon, Richard, 61
No-fault divorce, 11
Nonresearch registries and databanks,
    89-90
Norgay, Tenzing, 216-217
Nucleic acid sequence based amplification
    (NASBA) process,
    patent for, 202
Nucleotides, xiii

Oligonucleotide patents, 210
Olmstead precedent of 1928, 61
Omenn, G. S., 119
On the Origin of Civilization (Whately), 135
Orange (CA) County Superior Court,
    Calvert case and the, 33
Origin of Species (Darwin), 132
Owen, David, 218

Panelli, Edward A., 34
Paris Convention, 195
Parkinson's disease, 109
Partial sequences, patenting of, 204
Patent Cooperation Treaty, 186
Patent protection in the United States
    biotechnology and genetic engineering
        patents, 190-192
    discovery vs. invention, 187-189
    genetic testing and manipulation,
        185-187
    intellectual property and genetic
        testing, 181-198, 199-208, 209-214
    manipulation of plants and animals,
        189-190
    NIH cDNA patent applications,
        192-194, 199, 200, 215-216, 217-218
    patents for DNA sequences, 209-214
    patent system and U.S. competitiveness,
        195-196
    policy issues, 194-195
    scope and value of, 177-179

Patient autonomy, 49-50
Pearson, Karl, 136, 137
Pedigree studies, 89-92
Pelagius, 166
Pharmaceutical industry and the patent
    system, 191-192
Phenylketonuria (PKU), 106
Plant patents, 189-190
Plant Variety Protection Act, 189, 191
Plato, 132
Plomin, Robert, 121
Political level, privacy at the, 54-55
Polygamy, 9, 10
Polymerase chain reaction (PCR), patent
    protection for, 186, 202, 203
Popper, Karl, 155
Population genetics, 136-142
Prediction through genetics, 48-49
President's Commission for the Study of
    Ethical Problems in Medicine
    and Biomedical and Behavioral
    Research, 92
Prison population in the U.S., 147
Privacy
    breach of, civil suits for, 97
    definitions, 78-79
    and genetic information, 49, 53-100
    issues of, 17-21
    privacy rights, the foundation of, 81-82
Probe fragment, 200
Prospective Queer Parents, 40
Protestant Reformation, 166
Public policy needs and the family, 37-39
Punishment and blame, 158
Purkinje cells, 111
Purpura, Dominick, 107-108

Quantitative trait locus (QTL) method, 115

Rabuzzi, Kathryn Allen, 19
Randomly amplified polymorphic DNA
    (RAPD) technique, patent for, 202
Reaction norm, concept of, 115
Receptor diversity, 109
Recombinant DNA techniques, 201-202
Recombinant drugs/vaccines, patented,
    200-201

Reductionism and responsibility, 123-124
Registries, genetic, 85-86
  nonresearch registries and databanks,
    89-90
Reid, Thomas, 171
Religion within the Limits of Reason Alone
  (Kant), 168
Religious ethcists on germline
  enhancement, 220-221
Republic, The (Plato), 132
Reserve, 56
Responsibility
  and determinism, 171-172
  and reductionism, 123-124
Restriction enzymes, 202
Retardation, 119
  mental illness and mental retardation,
    156
Rights of informational self-determination,
  83-89
Rougement, Denis de, 13
Rowe, David, 142
Russell, Bertrand, 20-21

Schizophrenia, 109, 117-118
"Sequence-tagged sites," 107
Sexual psychopath statutes, 159
Short-sleep (SS) lines, 118
Sickle-cell anemia, 164
Single-parent families, 11
Smith v. Jones, 33
Social equality, genetics and, 162-165
Social policy and family
  relationships, 9-23
Sociocultural level, privacy at the, 55-56
Solitude, 56
Somatic therapy, 219-220
Southern blot procedure, 202
Spencer, Herbert, 133, 134
Sperm donors, 31
Stanford-Binet tests, 121, 139
Stanford University, 185
State University of New York (SUNY), 200
Sterilization, 144-146
Stern, Bill, 32, 35
Strong, Augustus, 166-167
Substance abuse, 117

Suffolk (NY) County Court, genetic
  fingerprinting case, 17
Surrogate motherhood, 32
Surveillance, disclosure and, 57-58
Sutcliffe, Gregor, 107

Tagged genes, 107
Tarasoff case, 50
Tay-Sachs disease, 12, 17, 164
Tennant, F. R., 167
Terman, Lewis, 145
Tertullian, 166
Texas Medical Center, Houston, 221
Theological ethicists on germline
  enhancement, 220-221
Top-down strategies, 124
Trasler, Gordon, 123
Treatise of Human Nature (Hume), 168
Turkheimer, Eric, 114, 115

Ulysses's strategy, 95
Unification Church, 13
Uniform Parentage Act, 31, 35
United Church of Christ, 220
United Kingdom's Medical Research
  Council (MRC), 218
United Nations Universal Declaration of
  Human Rights, 20
United Nations World Intellectual
  Property Organization (WIPO), 218
United States. *See also* Patent protection in
  the United States
  American public opinion about
    privacy, 64-65
  current privacy environment, 62-64
  infant mortality rate, 141
  new privacy expectations and rules,
    60-62
  prison incarceration rates by race
    in the, 147
  privacy crisis of the 1960s, 59-60
U.S. privacy tradition, 1787-1945, 58-59
U.S. Code, Title 35 of the, 183, 197-198
U.S. Code of Federal Regulations,
  Volume 37 of the, 183
U.S. Congress, new immigration laws, 145

U.S. Constitution
  Article 8, 177, 187, 194
  First Amendment, 59
  Fourth Amendment, 61-62
U.S. Department of Energy, xiv, 68
U.S. Patent and Trademark Office (PTO),
    177, 188
  In re Chakrabarty, 190
  intellectual property and the, 183
  on plant patenting, 189
  ruling on NIH cDNA patent
    application, 215-216
U.S. Public Health Service (PHS), 86
U.S. Supreme Court
  on Barefoot case, 156
  on capital punishment of children and
    the mentally ill, 158
  on Moschetta case, 36-37
  and privacy issue, 61, 62-63
University of California, 185
  State Oath of Allegiance and Patent
    Agreement, 205
University of Utah, 200
"Use," definition of, 184, 200, 204
Use patents, 203, 205
Utilitarianism, 19

Valuing and measuring, 163-164
Variable number of tandem repeat (VNTR)
    locus, 200
Venter, J. Craig, 107, 216
  NIH filings, 193-194, 215
Vermont's adoption law, 40
Violence, 148-149
  genetics, crime, race, and, 146-148
Violence and Traumatic Stress Research
  Branch, 148

Virginia
  incarceration rates by race in, 147
  involuntary sterilization bill, 145
Virginia Declaration of Rights, 125

Watergate incident, 61
Watson, James D., 124, 216, 217
Weber, Max, 20
Weissman, Myrna, 11
Wesley, John, 166
Westin, Alan, 82
Whately, Richard, 135
Whitehead, Alfred North, 19
Whitehead, Mary Beth, 32-33, 38
White House Office of Science and
    Technology Policy (OSTP) Gene
    Patent Working Group, 216
White, Ray, 17, 200
Wilson, Edward, 142
Wilson, James Q., 142
Wittgenstein, Ludwig, 135
Women
  families headed by, 11
  and monogamy, 10
Working Group of the European
  Community, 4
World Council of Churches, 16, 220
World Intellectual Property Organization
    (WIPO), 183, 186, 218

XYY factor, 146-148
  and criminality, 121-122
XYY males, 146-147, 156-157

Yeast artificial chromosome (YAC),
    186-187

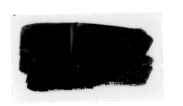